GRACEFULLY YOU

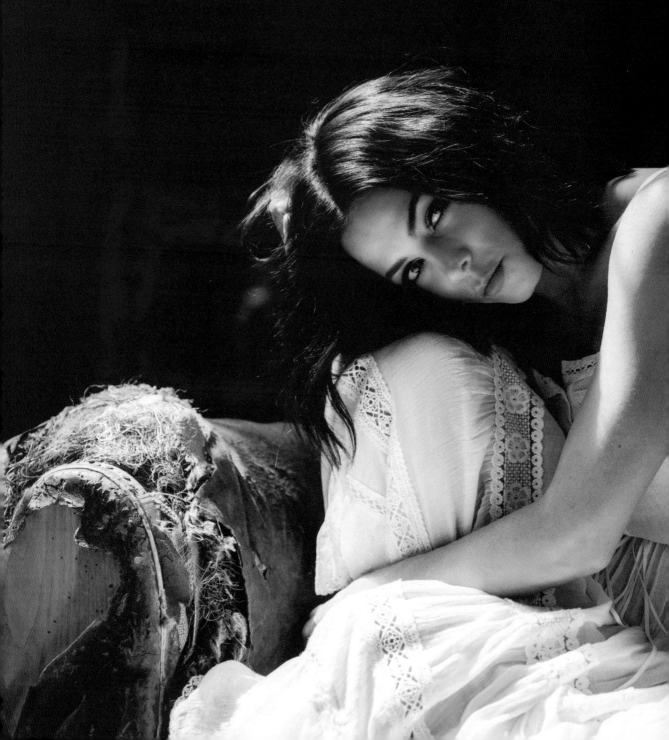

Gallery Books
An Imprint of Simon & Schuster, Inc.
1230 Avenue of the Americas
New York, NY 10020

First Gallery Books hardcover edition October 2019

GALLERY BOOKS and colophon are registered trademarks of Simon & Schuster, Inc.

For information about special discounts for bulk purchases, please contact Simon & Schuster
Special Sales at 1-866-506-1949 or business@simonandschuster.com.

The Simon & Schuster Speakers Bureau can bring authors to your live event. For more
information or to book an event, contact the Simon & Schuster Speakers Bureau at
1-866-248-3049 or visit our website at www.simonspeakers.com.

Interior design, lettering, and illustrations by Jane Archer @psbellanyc | janearcher.nyc
Interior photographs by Cory Tran

Manufactured in the United States of America

10 9 8 7 6 5 4 3 2 1

Library of Congress Control Number: 2019944815

ISBN 978-1-5011-9151-0
ISBN 978-1-5011-9153-4 (ebook)

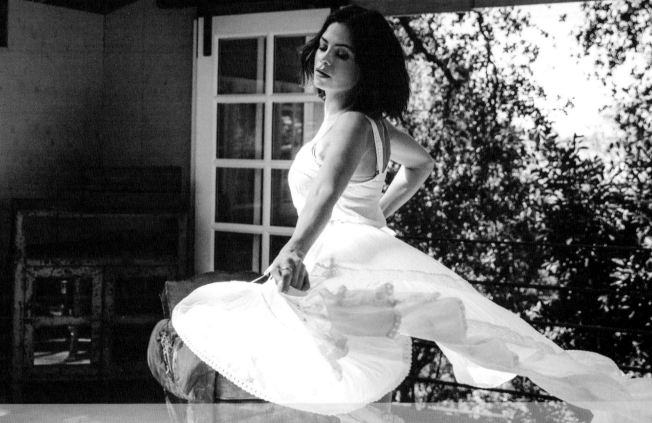

GRACEFULLY YOU

finding beauty and balance in the everyday

JENNA DEWAN

with ALLIE KINGSLEY BAKER

GALLERY
BOOKS

NEW YORK   LONDON   TORONTO   SYDNEY   NEW DELHI

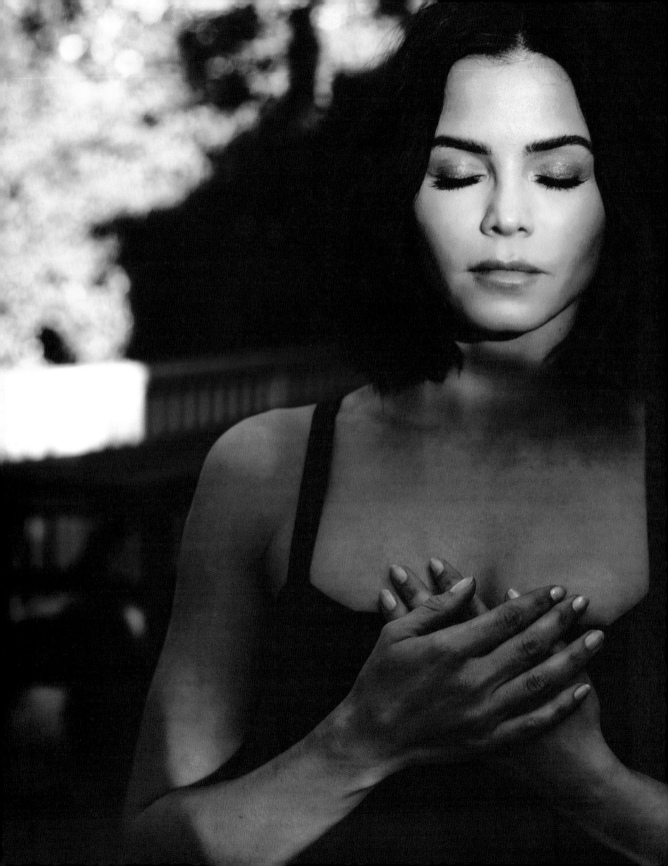

To my little fairy,

EVIE.

May you always

know your magic.

contents

1 INTRODUCTION

CHAPTER ONE:
9 *Live Awake*

CHAPTER TWO:
45 *Sacred Space*

CHAPTER THREE:
77 *Inner Beauty Rituals*

CHAPTER FOUR:
107 *Plant Life*

CHAPTER FIVE:
135 *Very Personal Style*

CHAPTER SIX:
151 *Body Work*

CHAPTER SEVEN:
175 *Mind Your Business*

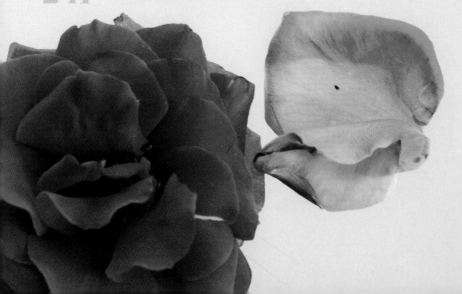

CHAPTER EIGHT

193   *Little Goddesses*

CHAPTER NINE

213   *Gracefully You*

237   CONCLUSION: GRACEFULLY NOW

241   ACKNOWLEDGMENTS

it is not only

time

which heals the soul:

it is presence

and patience

and faith

and creativity

and silence

and solitude

and breathing

(just breathe)

it is reconnecting with the things

which feed your soul—

the things which bring you back to your soul.

for it was you who wandered . . .

but you are coming home now.

                                              —APRIL GREEN

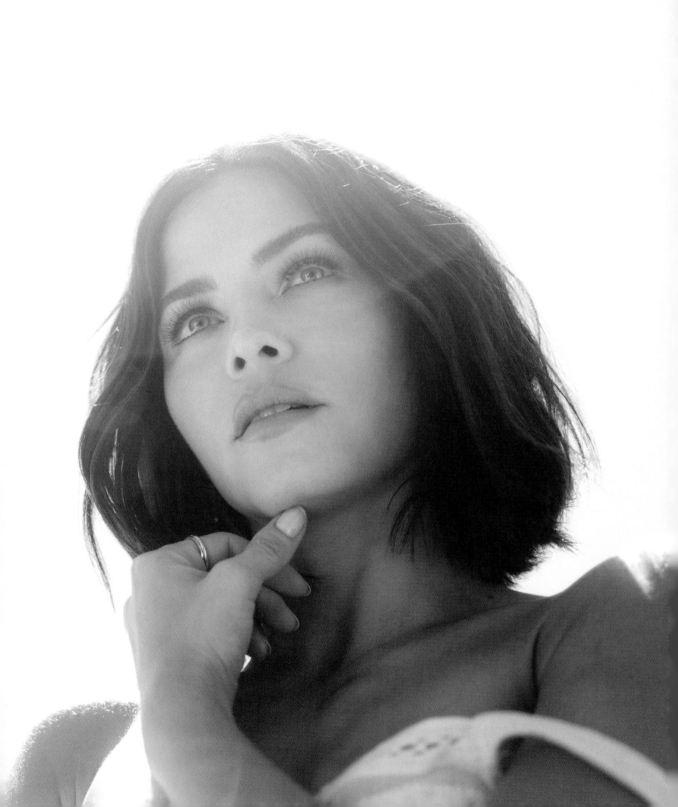

f rom a very young age I felt mystified by and drawn to the idea of finding a connection to something bigger than myself. My parents were neither religious nor spiritual. They didn't teach me to believe in a higher power or anything along those lines. Yet I still felt it was my calling to discover the magical presence in the universe I knew existed.

When I began dancing at age five I felt my first inkling of this powerful presence. I'd walk onto the stage and something behind my eyes would change–through dance I could throw myself into a foreign mindset, channeling an energy that was beyond my own. I had a strength, confidence, and fierceness onstage that was different from how I felt in my day-to-day life. They used to call me Little Tornado! Dancing gave me an immediate link to something I could feel. It was my passion that showed me how it felt to be connected to something bigger than myself, and this magical feeling has stayed with me throughout my life. When I'm dancing for myself or performing for others is when I feel the most connected to the energy. I feel lit up from the inside, completely in control, and very much in the flow of life.

When I was twenty-one, dancing on tour for Janet Jackson, I developed a friendship with the on-tour masseuse. We spoke at length about spirituality, which I was interested in learning more about and which she was well versed in. At the end of the tour, the masseuse gave me a beginner's book on chakras. It was my first introduction to the centers of energy that live inside us. I felt an immediate sense of déjà vu, as if I was remembering something I have always known. Learning about the seven chakras instilled in me an insatiable curiosity

regarding all things spiritual. I spent years devouring book after book, visiting Reiki masters, energy healers, and angel workers. I would lie on crystal beds in Topanga Canyon, participate in ceremonies led by shamans, and experiment with traditional spiritual medicines. I was constantly exploring, in search of a way to experience the same magic I was able to feel when I was dancing, but in all aspects of my life.

My curiosities led me on a life-changing trip to Peru for a charity organization I had been working with. I spent time deep in the Amazon with a tribe, living as they did. I found myself in awe of and inspired by the way the group's members connected to life, which was through nature. It was in stark contrast to what I was used to, even though I've always considered myself a nature lover. For most of us, we go on a hike and we pass by a tree or a flower and we think, *Wow, that's pretty.* The members of this tribe stop and pay respects. They'll say, "This tree is special because it is used for this and that. And that flower over there has great healing properties. It can be used for this and that." For them, there is no passing by anything in nature without acknowledging its relationship to us. This way of being opened my eyes and brought me to a spiritual turning point. I always considered myself someone who respects and appreciates the science and beauty of Mother Nature. But it wasn't until I stepped out of my mind-set and spent time with this tribe that I understood that in order to achieve a deep connection with ourselves, we also have to connect deeply with nature.

Returning home from Peru, I felt a strange combination of conflicting emotions. On one hand I felt extreme culture shock at being back in the hustle and bustle of my regular life. On the other I felt protected by a buffer, having been cocooned by the soothing sounds of the birds and a peace that only exists in a secluded jungle. The very next day after my trip, I had to present at the American Music Awards in Los Angeles–pretty much the antithesis of where I'd been. After my glam team put the final touches on my hair and makeup, I stepped into a glittering dress and turned to face a mirror. I gasped, taken aback by the shock of my transformation. I hadn't even taken a shower three days prior to arriving back home. Just when I had adjusted to living the sweaty green plant life, boom–there I was in a dress with a plunging neckline, about to hit the red carpet. And that's the balance that works for me. I don't want to live forever in the jungles of Peru, nor do I want a sparkling Hollywood life all the time either. I believe you don't have to be 100 percent this or that. You can be in touch with nature and connect to a spiritual presence while also shopping for manufactured moisturizer–instead of rubbing saffron on your cheeks. It's all about balance.

When it comes to living in that flow of energy we all love and strive for, to achieve the feeling of *I'm so grateful and joyful and life is supporting me*, I've learned that ultimately it all comes down to a few simple things: the personal bond you have with yourself, the relationship you have with nature, and your connection to a greater presence. With this realization I stopped questing outside of myself for what would make me feel connected and started going inward. I now know that when you stop searching outwardly and start looking and working within is when you learn who you truly are and understand what it is you need and want in order to live your best life. I fully understand not everyone has the ability to pack up for Peru in search of self-expansion (or interest in doing so). Knowing this is what inspired me to write this book. I've been fortunate to have access to people and places that have encouraged me to open up and have taught me a great deal. In the chapters ahead I look forward to sharing this with you. Moving forward, you'll find a collection of rituals, meditations, recipes, mantras, and more that I use to connect to myself, to loved ones, and to the energy shared by us all. My hope is that each page will make you feel lighter and brighter, ready to take on anything that comes your way with positivity and grace.

Attachment

I can tell you that your soul will shatter into a
million pieces (which may take years to put back
together) if you keep holding on to cold hearts in the
hope that they will eventually become warm in your
hands.

—APRIL GREEN

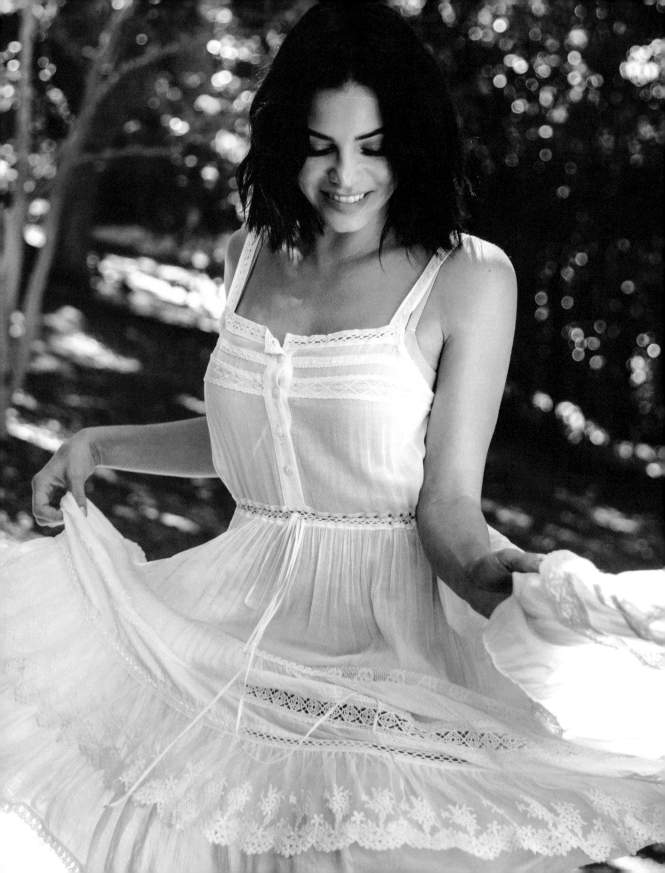

CHAPTER ONE

live awake

The most important part of my everyday begins with setting my intentions. This practice honors the desires I have for myself. Addressing these goals daily keeps me accountable and on track. For example, I might tell myself, *Today I intend to see the silver lining of every situation.* Am I able to control how the day will go? No. But I can establish early on how I plan to approach anything that comes my way. Chances are I'll face a disappointing reality, whether it's something major, like not landing a role I really wanted, or something small, such as a restaurant being out of what I planned on ordering. Since I made the commitment that day to see the silver lining, I will honor myself by finding the positive in every scenario. Living with this type of intention puts you in the driver's seat rather than leaving you at the mercy of life. It gives you the power to create not how the day will affect you but rather how you will effect the day. When I began living with this mind-set, my life completely changed for the better. I've come to accept that we are never in control of what happens around us; however, we can always take the reins on how we choose to feel about, react to, and move forward from events. Once you can harness and claim that power, I'm telling you, everything changes!

I decide first thing in the morning what I want my day to feel like. There's a difference between setting the expectation for how I want the day to go and deciding how I want to feel. It's important to focus on how you want to feel and not on what you want to happen. A lot of times people focus on things like *I intend to get that job* or *I intend to win that race*. At the end of the day, you can't control things like that, and you're only setting yourself up for potential disappointment. What you can control is the feeling you'll have going into it. For example, *I intend to feel confident* or *I intend to feel strong*. If I decide my intention for the day is to feel accomplished, it's going to affect the course of my day, no matter what. Say, for example, I get an enticing last-minute invitation to happy hour. I know the new plan will prevent me from going to my last meeting of the day. I'll stop to ask myself, *What will make me feel more accomplished: meeting up with my friend or making sure I meet that person for a potential work opportunity?* And the choice is simple, because I will immediately see what aligns with my intention for the day. If life happens and I have to pick up my daughter early from school, preventing me from taking my meeting, I'll still feel accomplished, but in a different

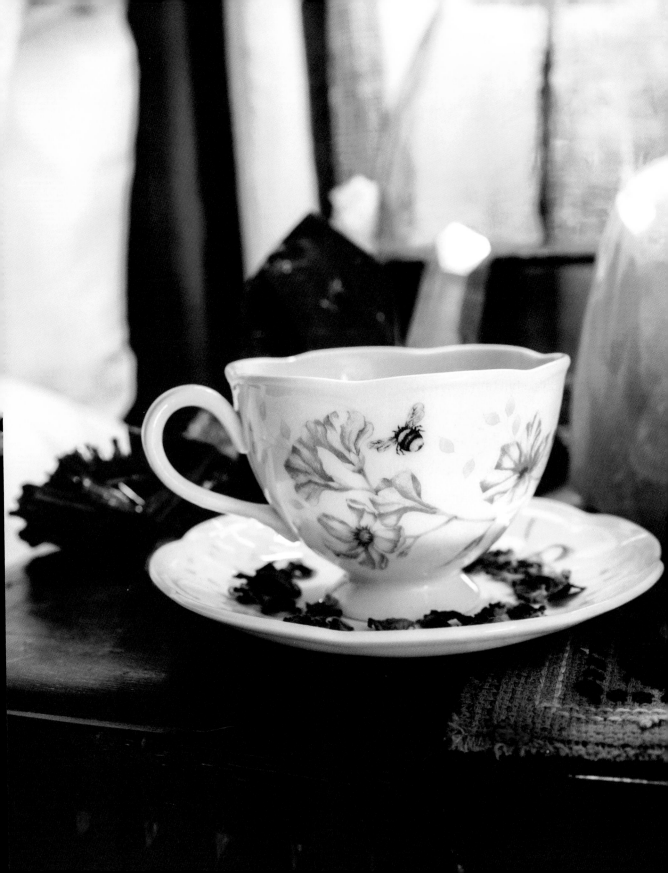

way. I will have accomplished my duty of being a dependable mom.

Setting your intention for each day is a small, easy thing to do, and it will make a huge difference in how you face each day. It made a huge difference in my life, and I have no doubt it will do the same for you!

In this chapter, you'll explore the practices and rituals I do every day that help me set an intention, feel a connection to the present moment, and connect to myself. Both the brain and the body respond positively to a sense of ritual. These little moments when I make time for myself have a big impact on my well-being, not only on a daily basis but in my life as a whole.

RISE AND SHINE
light shower

Taking even just five minutes to meditate first thing in the morning doesn't always seem possible when you've got kids wanting waffles, school drop-offs are imminent, or there's work waiting for your attention. But if your little one is anything like Everly, who is basically a barnacle on my body, the one place she won't follow you into is the shower. So the shower becomes a space that allows for a window of personal time to mentally and spiritually prepare for the day to come. It's where I like to combine a morning rinse with my meditation. Taking a shower is something I would do anyway, so why not take advantage of the precious time? If you think about it, the shower is an ideal place to create your own fantasy environment. It's warm and rejuvenating, and you're enveloped by the sounds of rushing water. You're able to pretend you're anywhere you want to be. I like to imagine I'm bathing in a secluded waterfall in the tropics. Cue the Enya.

Before you step in, imagine the showerhead is filled with a bright white liquid light. White represents positive energy. I think of the light pouring from the spout enveloping my body, cleaning off any stress and replacing it with love, happiness, strength, and positivity.

Once you're in the shower, close your eyes and breathe.

Focus on your breath and where it goes. Can you feel it in your chest? Does it fill your belly? If your back has been aching, send your breath there. Send each deep, intentional breath wherever you feel it needs to go.

Pay close attention to every drop of water as it rains upon your flesh. Feel it rolling off every part of your body.

Imagine the water is taking anything that doesn't serve you with it. Self-doubt, tension, or worry is washing away, streaming its way down the drain. Allow the water to strip you of any toxic or negative thoughts as they come to mind.

When you step out of the shower, know you are lighter, brighter, clean, and pure from the inside out. You're officially a clean slate.

As you dry off, set your intention for how you'd like to feel that day. Feel free to choose from one of my favorite go-tos: strong, in charge, decisive, accomplished, empowered, happy, relaxed, fearless, enthusiastic, proud.

oracle cards

Divination has been used and practiced for ages, by different cultures all around the world. The act of consciously connecting with a bigger presence through a specific modality is not a new age principle. Whether it was watching plants, reading the bones of animals that had been hunted, studying tea leaves impressions, runes, tarot . . . the list goes on. These beautiful cards have always spoken to me. They can be a guidance tool offering insight into any aspect of life, including relationships, health, careers, and so on. I use them as another means of living more intentionally. Anyone who knows me knows I always keep my cards nearby. They're usually next to or near my bed or in my bathroom. Sometimes I'll focus on an area where I could use a little insight or even ask a specific question as I'm pulling a card. Other times, I'll leave it up to the cards to decide what they'll bring me. I'll ask the cards, *What do I need to know for today?* To benefit from the cards, you don't have to believe in angels, spirits, or even the cards for that matter. At the very least, consider them flash cards of a type meant to inspire deep thoughts that allow you to get to know yourself a little better. It's not magic, but I do believe there is something deeper inside me that is actually selecting a card that speaks the most to me. Every morning I look forward to seeing what my unconscious wants me to bring my attention to.

Every card is different in its message. Some will contain an affirmation, and others will make you go a little deeper. They all provide a glimpse into your true self. You'll never pick a card and think, *That was random*. Every card will provide an answer to or insight on your innermost questions. The cards never teach me something I didn't already know on some level. They're not to be confused with a crystal ball or anything along those lines. They just allow me to access something I otherwise might not be considering or tapping into. They also often provide an extra boost of confidence when it comes to decisions I'm making.

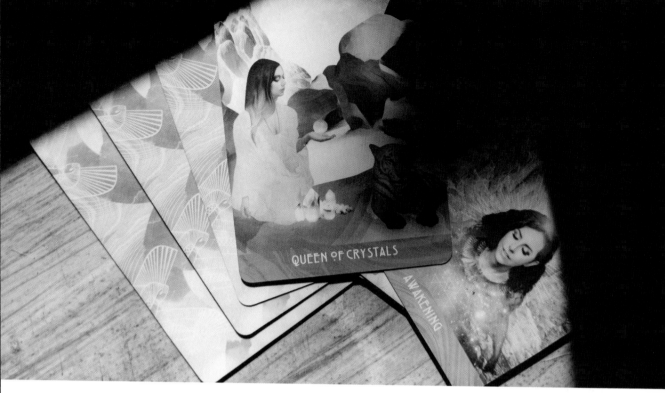

QUEEN OF CRYSTALS

AWAKENING

Everly gets beyond excited when she's able to pull her own card. I do my best to explain the cards to her in a way she can relate to, something a little deeper than just "Look, Mom, it's the purple unicorn card!" Once after reading her card she asked me, "How can my heart be even bigger today? What does that mean?" This inspired a memorable conversation about ways she could be even kinder that day and the importance of doing something nice for others. My heart burst as I witnessed Everly's early experience of looking within herself and taking the opportunity to grow from it.

Checking in with the cards is a nice thing to do at the beginning of the day or even at the end. It's a way to quiet the noise of life, check in with yourself, and bring yourself inward. I enjoy surrendering to the cards in order to let them channel me into one direction of focus. It's very different from blindly meditating or sitting alone with my thoughts, because the cards will help me organize my mind a bit and guide me to where to send my thoughts. Working with them feels as if I am cocreating with life instead of just letting life happen to me.

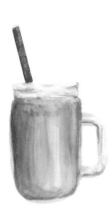

When it comes to nutrition, I've always felt that the first thing I put into my body is the most important. It took me a while to identify what my go-to breakfast would be. I am always on the go and busy; I wanted to find a meal I looked forward to having each morning that would benefit my body, but also something quick to make and easy to take with me. Some days I'll have time to whip up an avocado toast or oatmeal with berries, but most of the time, I just need to grab and go. All my nutritional prayers were answered when I came across a recipe created by my friend clinical nutritionist Kimberly Snyder. Not only is her Glowing Green Smoothie designed to benefit the body in so many ways (giving you clearer skin, smoother digestion, and renewed energy, among other things), but it's insanely good! My skin brightened up and my energy levels spiked almost immediately. I now make these smoothies at the start of every week and put them in the fridge. I pour each serving into a mason jar, write the date down on a label, and feel good knowing they're there right when I need one. I grab one first thing in the morning whether I'm running out the door or heading for the couch. I truly feel lit up when I'm drinking it, knowing I've already made the absolute best choice for my body and the day has only just begun!

glowing green smoothie

MAKES APPROXIMATELY 7 CUPS

$1\frac{1}{2}$ *cups water*

1 head organic romaine lettuce, chopped

3 to 4 stalks organic celery

$\frac{1}{2}$ *large bunch or* $\frac{3}{4}$ *small bunch of spinach*

1 organic apple, cored and chopped

1 organic pear, cored and chopped

1 organic banana, sliced

Juice of $\frac{1}{2}$ *fresh organic lemon*

OPTIONAL: $\frac{1}{3}$ *bunch organic cilantro (stems okay) and* $\frac{1}{3}$ *bunch organic parsley (stems okay)*

For my own personal touch, I like to add a scoop of spirulina, a plant-based source of protein, minerals, vitamins, and antioxidants.

Add water and chopped head of romaine to blender. Blend at low speed until smooth.

Add spinach, celery, apple, and pear, and blend at high speed.

Add cilantro and parsley (which help leach heavy metals from your body) and continue blending at high speed.

Finish by adding banana and lemon juice, blending until the desired consistency is reached.

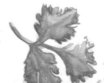

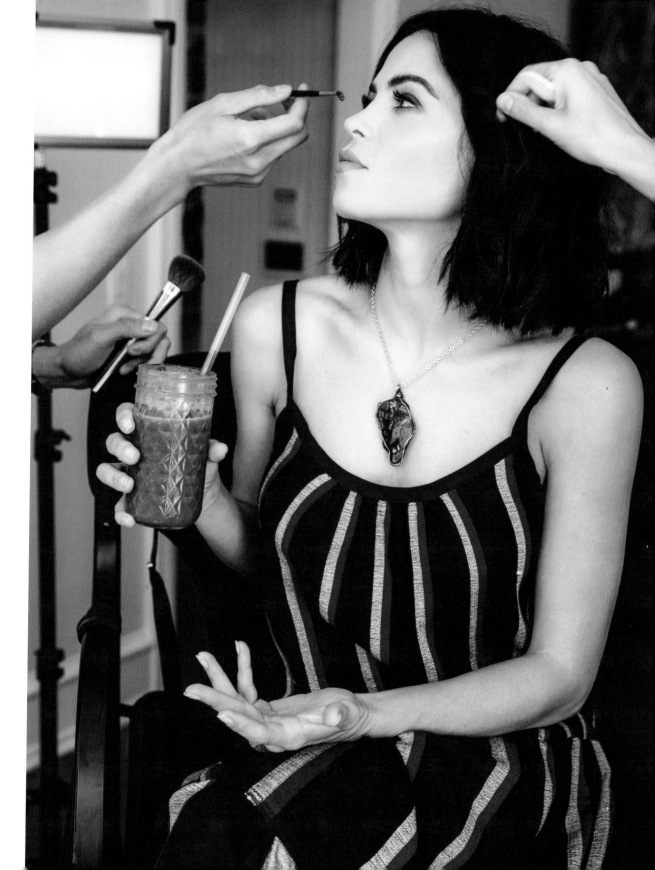

awakening stretch

For the sake of keeping it real, I don't always have time (okay, I'll keep it super real: I don't always remember) to work a moving meditation into my day. But when I do make the time, I am beyond grateful I did. A moving meditation is a chance to awaken your mind and body. More important, it is a way to connect your mind and body to each other. By going through these motions you're intentionally waking up your body while bringing your attention and thoughts inward. It's basically the best kind of multitasking there is.

Generally speaking, when I get overwhelmed or out of sorts it is because I have lost the connection with my body and therefore have stopped listening to and trusting what it's telling me. It is then that everything shoots up to my mind and seemingly gets stuck there. That's when I know I'm in trouble. Something magical happens when you slow down to acknowledge and activate each part of your body. Going through the emotions of an awakening stretch makes me feel connected, fired up, and ready to face whatever is in front of me. I learned the most effective moving meditation from my dear friend Scott Picard. I appreciate how Scott incorporates the elements of nature, earth, fire, water, and air into his meditation. Whenever I practice Scott's meditation I immediately see the value of myself. I instantly become a better version of myself. I find that I am more present, patient, and grounded. I feel connected to my body and feminine wisdom as a result.

Give this meditation a try and tell me you don't feel all the good things! Plan ahead by creating a private, quiet space for yourself. You won't need much room, since you'll be standing. You might want to read the meditation aloud and record it into your phone so you can play it back to follow along. Or if you have a friend who can spare seven or so minutes, have them read it to you. Either way, speak softly and slowly so you can take your time through the meditation. Take a momentary pause between paragraphs so you can settle into each movement.

Stand up in a natural, relaxed state. Allow your feet to melt into the floor. Close your eyes and begin.

Moving Meditation
Roll your eyes back and imagine they can roll all the way back. Let them travel down through your body. Imagine your eyes can travel all the way to your feet. Let all your attention go to your feet. Imagine your feet can spread wider as they sink into the earth.

Now start breathing through your feet. On the exhale, shoot breath into the earth through your feet. On your inhale, imagine you can bring your breath up just to the bottoms of your feet. In and out, you are shooting breath into and out of the earth through your feet.

Bring the breath up again just to the bottoms of your feet. Imagine now you can send roots from the bottoms of your feet into the earth. These roots extend all the way down, deep, deeper into the earth. The roots spread across the country, around the world. You're completely connected to the planet by your feet.

And now imagine the energy of the earth starts to travel up into your body. Like the wind, it moves up through your body.

Ask this question: *How is my body moved by the energy of the earth?* Allow your body to answer the question through movement. Allow your mind to relax and let your body answer through movement. Let yourself be moved by the earth.

Let the energy move into your heart. Imagine the energy moving effortlessly into your heart as you continue to breathe through your feet. Ask yourself: *How does the energy of the earth allow my heart to feel?* Imagine just showing with your body what the energy of the earth allows your heart to feel. Show this with movement.

Now I want you to imagine that deep within the earth is a fire. That fire goes up through your feet and into your legs. It's as if you're standing in the middle of a bonfire. Ask yourself: *How is my body moved by fire energy? What does fire energy give to my body?* Keep moving. Imagine the fire goes all the way into your heart. Ask yourself: *What does fire energy allow my*

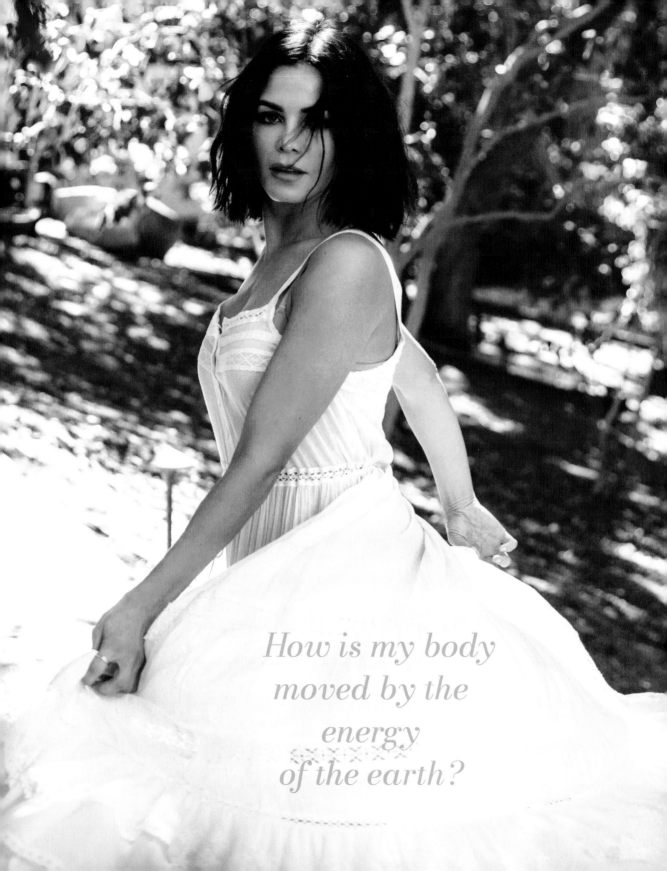

*How is my body
moved by the
energy
of the earth?*

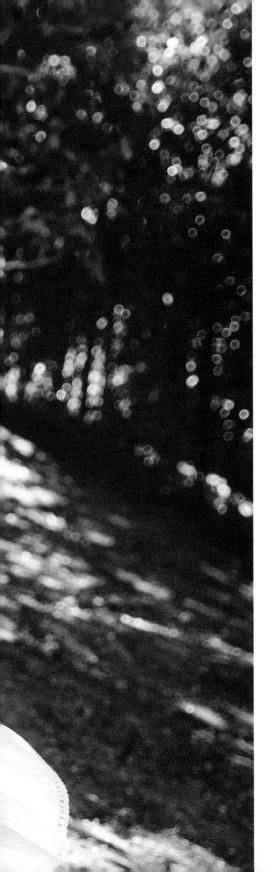

heart to feel? Imagine you're on a stage and you have to show everyone what it means to have fire energy in your heart. Let your body go and do whatever it wants to do.

Now let your eyes roll back and imagine they fall back into your belly. You find yourself floating on your back in the water that is in your belly as you connect to water energy. Ask yourself: *How does water move my body? How is my body moved by the energy of water as I float on my back in the ocean?* Feel the depth of the ocean beneath you, supporting you. Ask yourself: *What does water energy allow my heart to feel?*

As you stay lying on your back, spread your arms open like wings, pushing out your chest. Imagine the immensity of the sky can pour itself into your chest. Ask yourself: *What does air energy give to my body?* Imagine the sky continuing to pour itself into your heart. *What does air energy allow my heart to feel?*

Return to your stance and breathe the earth through your feet. Move the energy from the earth, connect it to the fire, and at the same time, connect to the water in your belly. Connect the earth, fire, and water to your upper body, which is air. You're now running all elements at the same time: earth, fire, water, and air. Let your body naturally move in these elements. Ask yourself: *If my human body was the one place where all these elements could move, dance, live, and work together, what could be possible in my life?*

Continue to move in all four elements. Ask yourself: *What is the person inside me learning?* Don't worry about answering with your mind, just move.

When you're ready, gently come out of the meditation.

SWEET DREAMS

D.R.E.A.M.

Disconnect
Reach
Evaluate
Ask Why
Meditate

Is there any better feeling than the exact second your head ever so softly hits the pillow and your entire body dissolves into the dreamy abyss that is sleep? Well, I know firsthand that it doesn't come that easily all the time. I was an incredible sleeper my entire life. I even slept through a massive earthquake as a kid while visiting my dad in San Francisco! I slept like a rock. That is, until my early twenties. I had just gotten off tour with Janet Jackson and was feeling the big-time anxiety of *What's next?* Dancing for Janet was my dream job at the time, and at twenty-one I had already accomplished my biggest goal! Also I was getting out of a relationship with a boyfriend who was mentally and emotionally manipulative. We were both young, he wasn't always up-front or honest with me, and I ignored all the red flags—you know how it goes. It was my first time experiencing the fallout of giving away my power and ignoring my own self-love in order to "be cool and fit in." It was a tough lesson.

The relationship ended quite dramatically with my sensitive heart feeling very confused and manipulated. Those thoughts and feelings, combined with the unknown reality of what my life would look like after ending the tour, led me to stop sleeping. I mean that quite literally—I just stopped sleeping. For a few months, I tossed and turned, paralyzed with anxiety for the first time in my life. I can now look upon this time in my life as a great lesson in self-love, and in beginning to master what every woman or man needs in life, and that is boundaries. You need to love yourself enough to not give away your energy to people who are not worthy. It took some time, therapy, healing, reading, spiritual work, and making new friends for me to get past that period, but the other side of pain is always worth it. Even though I still struggle with sleeplessness from time to time, especially during emotional times in my life, for the most part my sleeping became regular. One of the things that helps me a lot is to check off a few essential pre-slumber steps. Taking a few minutes to touch on these rituals makes sleepy time easier, more meaningful, and even sweeter. To keep myself accountable, I always try to remember that before I fall asleep I've got to D.R.E.A.M.

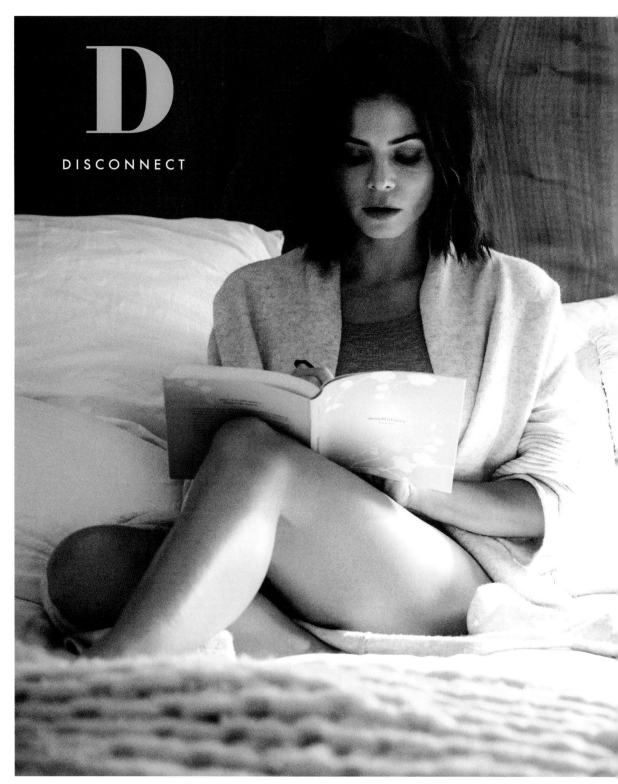

D

DISCONNECT

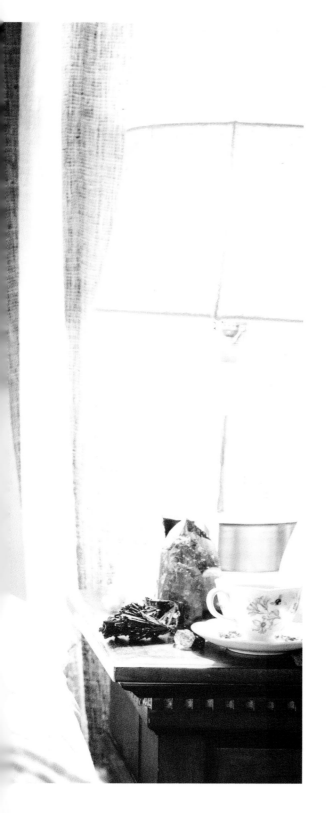

D = Disconnect

At least twenty minutes before bedtime I try my best to unplug from all things screen. I silence and put away my phone, computer, tablets—you get the idea. By unplugging from these distractions I allow myself to begin an inner dialogue of my own. Not to mention that by doing so you'll be avoiding the harmful effects of the artificial blue light emanating from our screens. It's been proven that blue light strongly suppresses the secretion of melatonin, the chemical that helps us fall and stay asleep. Now, if you are like me sometimes and just can't tear yourself away, I suggest turning on the nighttime light function on your phone and adhering to a no-social-media rule. Download an app that allows you to read and be introspective. I love the Alana Fairchild Rumi Oracle app. Sometimes during my wind-down I will use that app to read and soothe my mind (another great sleeping tool is to have your unconscious speak to you a bit before bed).

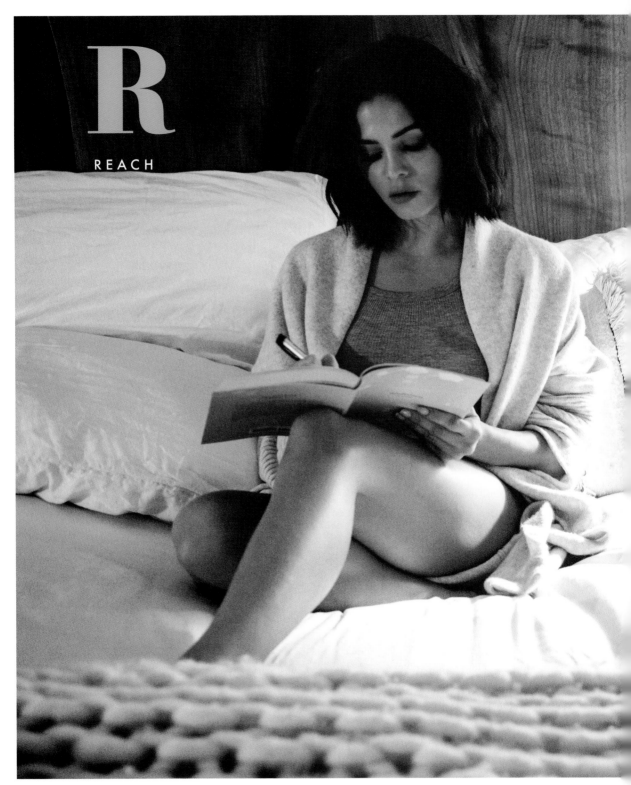

R

REACH

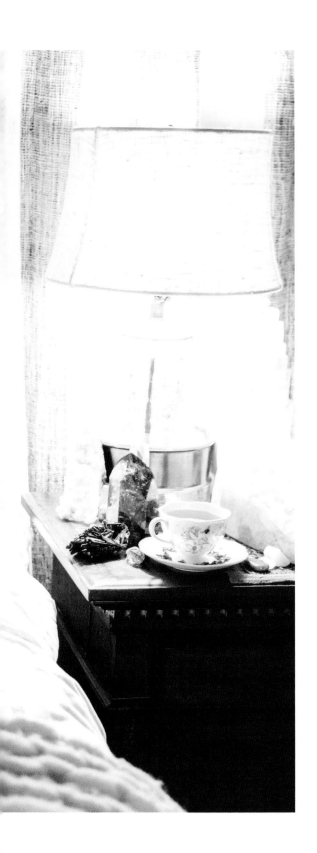

R = Reach

Give yourself a loving stretch from head to toe. Your body has worked hard today, so why not reward every inch? I like to start by wiggling my toes, rotating my ankles, pulling and stretching, making my way all the way up to my ears. Don't skip the smaller muscles like your fingers and jaw. Give each and every inch of your body a bit of attention before putting it to rest.

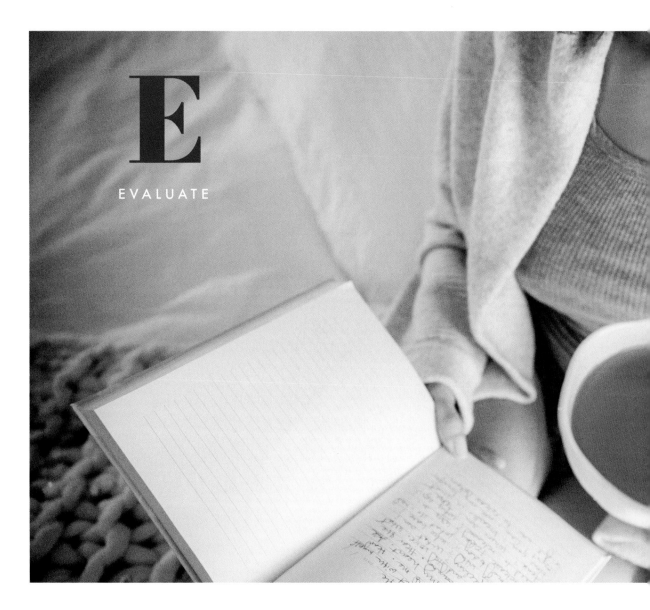

E

EVALUATE

E = Evaluate

Once I'm in bed I like to evaluate my day by journaling for five minutes. I try to journal every night, especially in times of crisis. I find that writing things down on paper is really the best way to get your feelings out of your mind. It's almost as if you're taking thoughts and worries off your chest and placing them elsewhere for the time being. I find this to be extremely liberating. It brings me a great sense of relief. I also believe it's good for your brain to go through what you've processed that day. It's like looking back

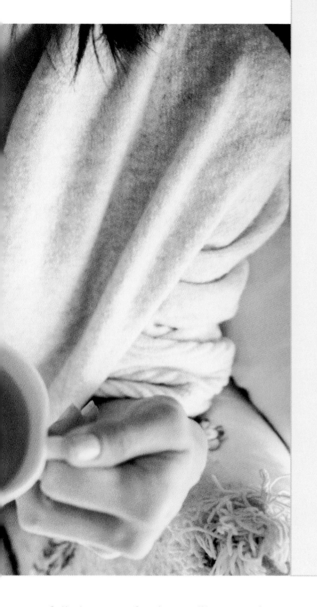

Words don't always flow as easily as I'd like them to. Sometimes I'll sit and stare vacantly at a blank page waiting for the words to magically appear. This can be especially frustrating. One thing that has helped me in this circumstance has been using prompts to get things going. For example, if you flip through my journal you'll find many of my entries start with "Today I felt . . ." This is a great way to instigate thought and emotion. After writing down how you felt that day, elaborate on why. Once you start to explain yourself, the pen will begin to wiggle, and before you know it, you'll be on your way to the next page.

on a full chapter of a day, pulling out the notable moments, identifying areas of growth, and recognizing experiences you had. You'll never regret taking the time to learn more about yourself.

I also love the idea that I'm creating a record I can look back on to see how far I've come. Sometimes I'll turn back to a few years ago and think, *Wow, I remember feeling my way through that, and I've come so far.* I would have loved to read my grandmother's journal from when she was my age to know what she experienced.

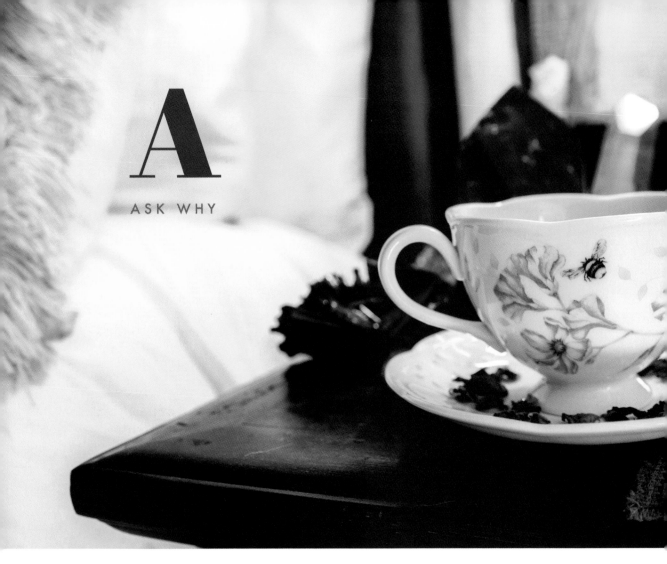

A

ASK WHY

A = Ask Why

On most days I feel very overwhelmed by life in general. Like you, I wear a lot of hats. I'm a mom first and foremost, but I also work on television shows and films, design for various brands, run a production company, do interviews, manage my house, and so on. I feel constantly pulled in a multitude of directions. Sometimes I get into bed and need to ask myself, *How are you feeling?* It's not every day, not even every week that someone asks you with complete sincerity, *How are you feeling?* It's very important to take honest stock of yourself.

On days like this my answer would be, "I'm feeling very overwhelmed." I then follow up with, *Why?* I might ex-

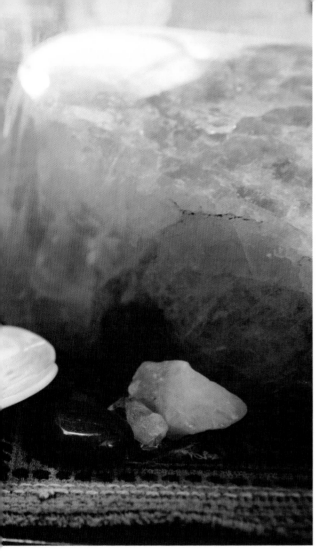

dig deeper. By asking myself why, I realized I'm not that overwhelmed—I just need to work on how I manage my time. This feeling I'm having doesn't have to last; in fact, it can easily be fixed. In most cases I've found the evaluation relieves the anxiety. This type of introspection shines a light on things that otherwise might be buried or hidden. By digging deeper, you'll ultimately get to a neutral place or learn to let negative emotions go.

It's incredible what we can learn and correct about our stressors if we just ask ourselves why. The "why" also works when it comes to recognizing the root of our positive feelings. If you say you're feeling loved and I ask why, perhaps you'll say it's because your partner makes you feel special. *Why?* They surprised you by washing your car. Why does that make you feel good? Because it makes you feel cared for and valued. It's important to identify what exactly makes us feel excited, loved, happy, stressed, and so on. Asking why forces us to go way beyond simply feeling an emotion.

plain by saying, "There were too many decisions that had to be made today." *Why?* "Well, I procrastinated." *Why?* "I wasn't taking time for myself, so I was putting off things I needed to do." *Why?* "I'm struggling with time management." Aha. By asking why, we can allow ourselves to surrender to the solution. The "why" is our shovel, which we can use to

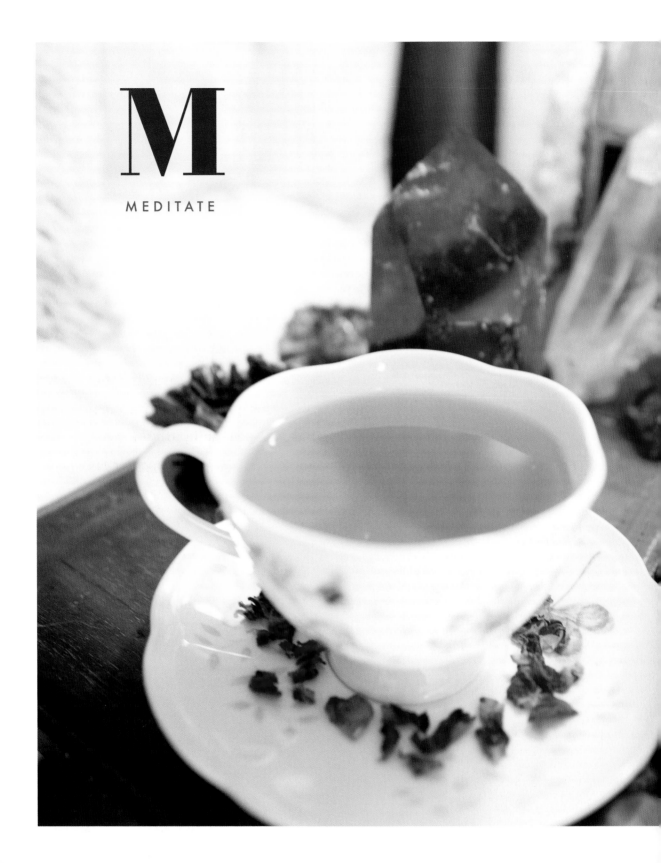

M

MEDITATE

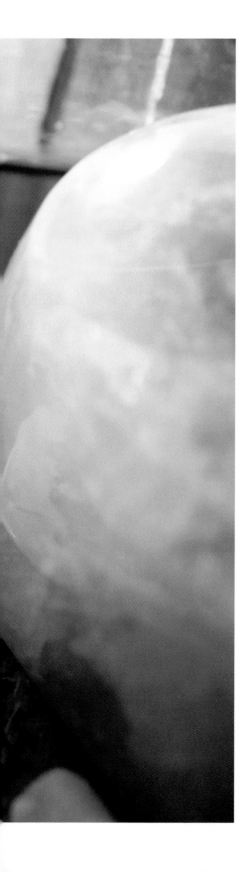

M = Meditate

Before I drift off to sleep I make it my intention to have the last thoughts on my mind be ones of gratitude and light. As I'm falling asleep, I try to think of three positive things, whether notable things that happened that day or something I'm grateful for. Even on a tough day when it's hard to find even one great moment, I'll focus on something simple I have to be grateful for, like my cozy pajamas, cool air-conditioning, or even my favorite song. I'm always grateful for my daughter, a warm bed, and the ability to move my body. It's the little things, the simple ones, that are sometimes the best.

refuel nights

Like you, I am BUSY. You might look at my Instagram feed and think, *Busy doing what?* I know it looks like I'm living a life of pure leisure when at 2 p.m. on a Tuesday I'm seen walking my dogs through a field for a post about athleisure wear. The reality is, that post is one of my job obligations and that photo was taken in my backyard, which I was in for maybe three minutes, in between meetings, calls, and racing to pick up my kid. We've all got our own kind of crazy going on—don't let the good lighting fool ya! That said, it's so easy for us to hit cruise control and go, go, go while burning the candle at both ends. *I've got to do this, have to hurry there, don't forget that, and back to this place before racing onward again.* It all feels so important and so overwhelming.

Sometimes I'll look at my calendar and think, *You've got to be kidding me!* While I'm grateful for a full life, I know that in order to maintain it, it's important for me to slow down and hit reset. You know the feeling you get when you've been going nonstop, the moment you hit a wall and wonder, *Why am I at empty?* I like to think of myself as a tank that needs gas. We need to constantly refuel ourselves. One thing I've gotten pretty good about is scheduling in a refuel night. If I see that I have a week full of events, photo shoots, and school plays ahead of me, I'll schedule in one night that week for a refuel.

On these nights, I'll put my daughter down and get into the headspace of *This is my time.* I may schedule an at-home acupuncture session or massage, or maybe I'll watch TV or read a book. But one thing I won't do is use my phone, and I especially won't go on social media. We live in a busy world, and even when we're not busy, we feel busy because we're looking at how busy other people are through our newsfeeds. When I'm trying to relax I don't want to witness someone else's great workout or watch them whip up a fantastic meal. It makes me feel guilty in that moment, like I should be doing more. Social media can make it seem like everyone else has a better balance in life, and it simply isn't true. I know people who don't have the easiest lives, but then I see them on social media and I think, *Wow, things look very different for them here.* It messes with the mind of the poster and with that of the viewer. Don't get me wrong, I'm certainly not anti–social media. But realize and understand that what you're seeing is everyone's "highlight" reel and keep it real.

There is a time and a place for scrolling, and for me, this place is not when I'm trying to come from a place of Zen, to maintain a relaxed state. Don't beat yourself up, though, if you find yourself having a hard time resisting. That doesn't help anyone! Start smaller, maybe by keeping away every other night, or on weekends, whatever you can do. Every little bit helps, and I promise you, when you feel the difference in your quality of sleep, you will be hooked!

In order not to hit a wall and thus force yourself into a time-out, you need to be a little bit ahead of the curve. Take a look at your schedule and recognize when you're going to be on and going for a stretch of time. This is when you know you'll need to schedule a refuel night. It might feel weird to book yourself for alone time. In a way, you have to be your own best friend. It's okay to look in the mirror and say, "Girl, you're going too hard and you need to take time for yourself. Stop giving out so much. Refuel your tank!" These refuel nights are really important. You deserve them.

In a way, you have to be your own best friend.

what to do on a refuel night

Keep your hands busy. If you find it challenging not to pick up your phone, don't let it be an option. I enjoy the simplicity of giving myself a manicure or even just painting my nails. It requires my full concentration, and there's the reward of having pretty hands at the end. For the same reasons, I also enjoy journaling.

Read in bed. I used to be a fanatical reader. When I was a kid I would read a book a day. I went through quite a depression when I was eleven after moving from Maryland to Texas. My mom was remarrying after it had been just her and me for a while, and I was leaving my beloved dance studio. I had made friends whom I felt very connected to, loved my life there, and was devastated to move. I had moved every three years as a kid, and in Maryland I had truly felt comfortable for the first time, that I was grounded and finding my groove. Let's just say it was a lot of change. While my mom was packing our life into boxes, I went to stay at our family house in Nantucket for two weeks with my grandparents. Being so young, feeling displaced, and not knowing what my new life would be like caused me to clam up. Everyone was worried because I was so quiet and withdrawn. Things changed one day when I found a bookstore I could ride my bike to. I'd pick up a book every morning and read one a day. I was big into YA mystery novels like the Nancy Drew and Hardy Boys series. But my favorite was The Baby-Sitters Club. I was obsessed and couldn't get enough of my favorite characters. I loved how every book was a new dilemma, an adventure they had to make their way through. I truly believe escaping through these books saved me from a deep depression. I created a special relationship with reading when I discovered how it switches off something in your brain. To this day, even if I'm just reading one chapter, it calms me through escape and distraction.

Watch a movie. On refuel nights, I'm all about the feel-good flicks, nothing stressful or scary. Give me laughter and light, all the rom-coms I can take! A few personal favorites: *Cry-Baby*, *Pretty Woman*, and of course *Dirty Dancing*.

Indulge in comfort food. My grandmother used to make me cinnamon-sugar toast. Having it now reminds me of what it felt like when my grandmother made it for me. It was a time I felt nurtured and loved. The scent and taste of this snack evokes those emotions for me. I'll show myself some care and comfort by making my grandmother's toast on my refuel night.

grandma's sweet toast

This snack is everything! It's also incredibly easy.

1. Butter a slice of bread.

2. Sprinkle on a pinch of cinnamon and a pinch of sugar.

3. Pop the topped bread into the toaster, broiler, or oven. Watch it closely to make sure it doesn't get too crispy or burnt!

4. Enjoy!

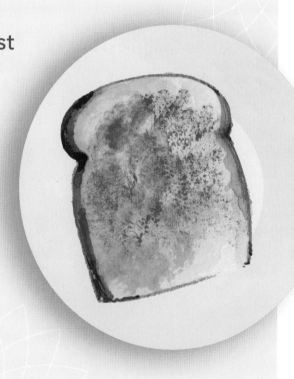

Drink calming refuel tea. When it comes to creating total relaxation, Mother Nature always knows best. I can't imagine a night of refueling without a cup of hot tea. I like to choose my herbs and spices based on what my intentions are. For example, if I've had a bit of a nervous stomach lately, I'll add a touch of fresh ginger. If it's pure unwinding I'm in search of, I'll reach for a kava or chamomile tea with a touch of lavender.

calming rose tea

MAKES 1 SERVING

This tea utilizes the natural properties of rose to calm and cool the body and mind. It promotes relaxation by reducing stress and calming the nerves all while promoting healthy, glowing skin.

2 cups filtered water
4 dried rosebuds or 2 teaspoons rose petals

In a small pot bring water to a boil. Add the rosebuds (or petals); reduce heat and simmer for 7 minutes. Remove from heat and strain out roses. Sip slowly.

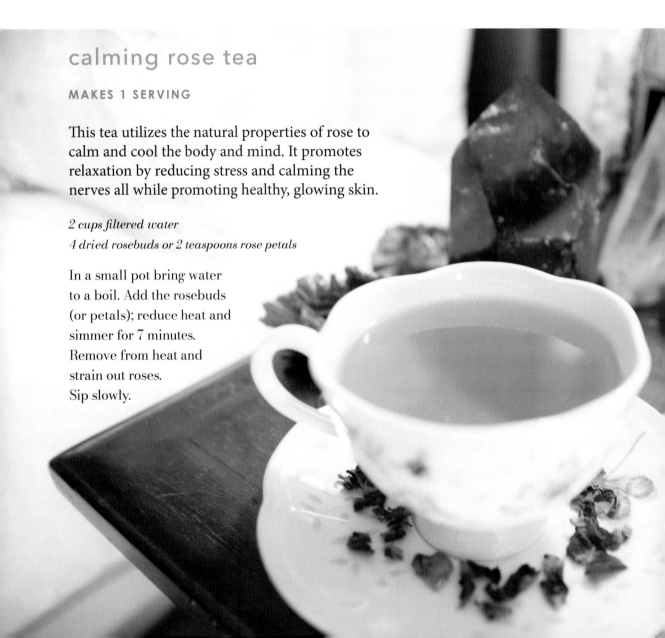

TAKE WITH YOU

Although I do my very best to begin and end each day with one or more of my rituals, the reality is, it doesn't always happen. And that's okay. Tomorrow is a new day, an opportunity to center myself and start fresh. The important thing to remember is to be positive, kind, and forgiving to yourself and to others. The rest will always fall into place.

no matter the pain

it has taken you to get here;

the love you have lost,

given up on (pass by).

the wars you have fought,

run from (chased after).

you are still the expanse of sky.

you are still the air,

the earth,

the moving tide,

and everything in between.

it is your birthright

to grow and ache

and change and learn

and hurt and heal.

love.

breathe.

you belong here.

— APRIL GREEN

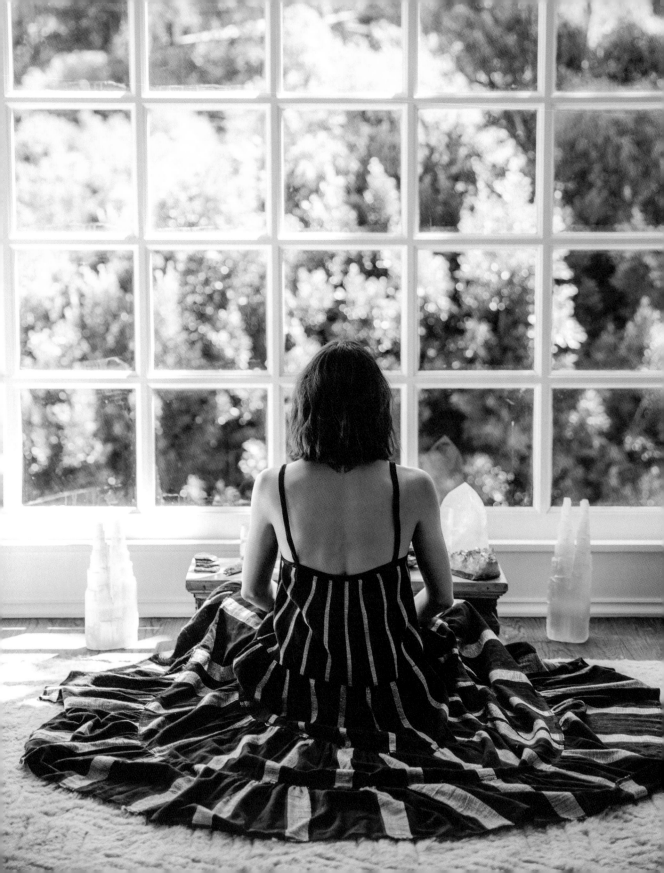

CHAPTER TWO

sacred space

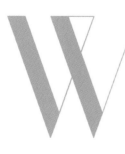hen it came to finding a place to call home, I knew exactly what I was looking for. I am one of those people who prefer wide-open spaces and bright, natural light. I wanted my home to feel like a deep breath of fresh air. I was ecstatic to find the house Evie and I now call home. Besides being spacious and free-flowing, it's surrounded by trees and lush landscaping. It was the

perfect canvas for us to color with our taste and imagination, making it our own.

Before I dove into decoration mode, I thought long and hard about what this new place would become for us. I considered what my priorities for each space would be. What type of home did I want to come home to? Comfort was of the utmost importance to me. I didn't want only the den to serve that purpose; rather, I wanted the whole house to be a place where people felt they could come together and relax. I didn't want a perfect and untouchable room, or even a precious corner. Everything in my house is something you can use, sit on, live in, and so on. I want every room to feel lived in and inviting: a sitting area that sucks you in and a dining space that lures you to the table. My goal is for anyone who stops by to feel a sense of lightness, love, comfort, and peace. Having that "wow factor" was never all

Little touches make all the difference when it comes to creating a meaningful environment.

that important to me. I don't need a grand foyer designed to impress. Besides, you can't really have a stuffy house with a five-year-old. I much prefer a home that feels deeply personal, one that is a true reflection of my energy and style.

My fashion sense and interior-design sense share a lot of similarities. I'd describe myself a lot of times as half hippie and half classic. In both aspects I gravitate toward comfortable yet feminine classic pieces. I appreciate a flowing bohemian dress just as much as I do a pair of jeans and sneakers. Like my wardrobe, my house has a lot of mixed textures and a laid-back personality. It looks very bohemian, but at the same time, it's grounded by clean lines and elevated taste.

Walking through my house you'll get a real sense of spirituality, because that's a part of who I am. In every room you'll find special crystals, meaningful statues, and books that are very reflective of what I am all about. It's important to me to surround myself with objects and art that speak to me, colors that encourage me, and collectibles from my travels or other moments that make me feel good. Yes, I realize that's a whole lot of "me." I believe these personal touches are what make a house a home, a sacred space to you and your family. If my house featured only generic, mass-manufactured things, it would look and feel like anyone lived there. Almost like a model home. Little touches such as framed photos or drawings by my daughter, sentimental gifts, and treasures that tell a story make all the difference when it comes to creating a meaningful environment.

I've learned you don't have to drop a mortgage payment to decorate if, like mine, your goal is to create a sense of warmth and welcome. One of my greatest treasures is a tea set my mom gave me that once belonged to my grandmother. Even though I am not a traditionalist like my mom and grandmother (in that I don't use or collect fine china, no matter how much they wish I did!), I still have this set on display. Every time I see it, I think of them. I much prefer this tea set to any other, knowing it was once enjoyed by the women in my family. I believe in objects rich with history, whether yours or someone else's. It gives that otherwise insignificant item a past and makes you feel good about being part of its story. I wish I owned more pieces like this. One of my favorite things to do is frequent flea markets and art fairs, where I can still find items with a past, things I know were once treasured and loved by someone else. These goods may not have been my grandmother's, but I like to think they once belonged to somebody's grandmother.

I find some of the coolest pieces this way. Once I came across a medium-size ornate tray. I brought it home and had Evie repaint it to make it her own. It became this really pretty thing, and I ended up placing it on a side table in the living room. Now guests often use it to hold their drinks, and they always comment on how unique it is. I love how this two-dollar find has become one of my most treasured items. As I have gotten older, I like the idea of surrounding yourself with things that once belonged to your family. It makes family members seem closer when they live far away, or even once they're no longer around. I've made it a priority to invest in meaningful things to be passed down to Evie, her children, and so on. For example, I commissioned a painting of Evie and me by an incredible Renaissance-style painter. Due to its large size and old-world style, it feels very significant, as I imagine an heirloom should. I love having it in our home, especially knowing its sentimental value will be passed down from generation to generation.

With all this collecting, you might imagine that my house resembles some kind of hoarder situation, but it's actually the complete opposite. It is not in my nature to be organized, so trust me when I tell you I have to work really hard to make my home that way! I routinely try to go through everything, constantly moving things out before anything additional moves in. I am very keen on Marie Kondo's method of letting go of clutter and keeping only what brings you joy. I strongly believe in energetic space, that your surroundings correlate with how your heart and brain feel. There's so much *stuff* that piles up (especially when you have a kid), and I always feel overwhelmed by the overabundance of these things. As bad as I am about letting these things pile up, I've learned to become just as good about letting them go. I try my best to routinely move out of our space things that are no longer serving us, whether that means giving books we've already read to a library, donating toys and clothes, or recycling the four nearly empty shampoo bottles I know I'm never going to finish (you know what I'm talking about).

I see a house as its own living, breathing being, a part of the family that needs as much love and care as those who live in it. While the house itself provides us with shelter, safety, and a sense of space, we make it a home by giving it energy, order, and light. I practice the following at-home rituals in order to maintain a high vibration of positive energy throughout our home.

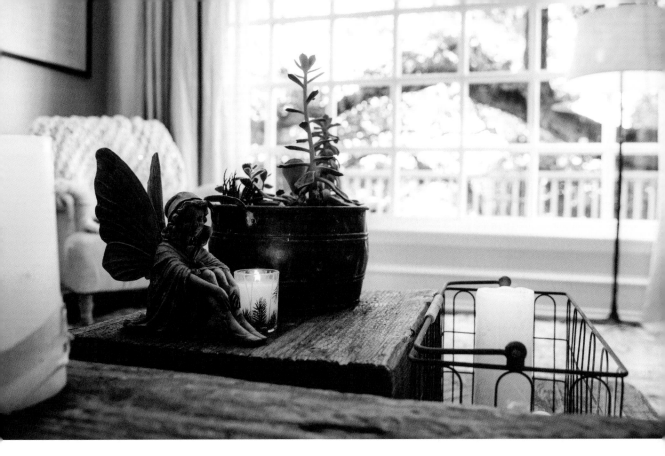

BON VOYAGE

Truth be told, I'm naturally a very messy person. Not for a second do I claim to be an organized, keep-it-all-together kind of girl; however, I do intentionally work hard to be better and to keep myself and my space in check. I used to shop—a lot. I'd pile clothes into my closet, things I just had to have in that moment. When I saw a cute shirt I liked, I'd buy one in every color. Why have one or two pairs of favorite jeans when you could have twenty? As I got older, I realized that less truly is more. I no longer shop for the sake of shopping. Instead, I save and wait to buy fewer splurge items as opposed to a roomful of space killers. In the end, I feel much better about a cleaner closet than I do about an overindulgent, cluttered room full of stuff. Besides, selecting an outfit of the day is much easier when you have a small number of options you love as opposed to a million things that are meh.

Have you ever noticed that when you're

feeling emotionally overwhelmed and chaotic, your living space seems to reflect that? When my mind is juggling thoughts and I'm feeling a bit scrambled internally, I've also got papers, bills, and notes piled around the kitchen, half-read books tucked into random corners, laundry still waiting to be put away, and an overall cluttered environment. To me, it is so blatantly obvious that our energy is reflected in our space! I believe that in order to get your mind right, you've got to get your house in order, too. If I'm feeling overwhelmed about anything, I'll take five minutes to pick up my physical space, and it will instantly do wonders for my mind-set and mood.

Doing mini-purges here and there in addition to two full-on clean sweeps a year forces me to be much saner. This has proven to be a real force against my messy side, which can otherwise easily take over. Since I've been practicing the art of living with less, I've honestly noticed a big differ-ence in my life.

Getting rid of stuff just feels so damn good. It really does. I've noticed a pro-found effect on my sleep and overall anx-iety. Even just the word itself, *stuff*, is so empty and meaningless. Who wants *stuff*?

Clearing your space of physical ex-cess isn't always about making room. Often it's about letting go of anything that brings you less than good vibes. If you've attached an upsetting memory or the thought of someone who hurt you to something—get rid of it. If you have a delicious-smelling candle that came from an ex and it still reminds you of your bad breakup every time you smell it, it's time to buy a new candle. Every time I've had a breakup, I've made the choice not to hold on to my former partner's things. I always give them back. Anything that brings you down even one decibel or impacts you negatively in any way—get rid of it. Sur-rounding yourself with positive memories and uplifting messages instead will make your space—and, in turn, you—feel much lighter and brighter. Having a clear space is essential for a fresh start, especially post-breakup. Sure, it can be difficult to part with those memories, but it is necessary for feeling the absolute finest in your sacred environment.

Some people believe in saving all their journals, but I had one journal in particular I felt had to go. I wrote in it during a time when I was really down on life, experiencing loss and deep heartache. The book felt so heavy to me, knowing it was filled with so much hurt and devastation. Having it in my space, even just knowing it existed, felt uncomfortable for me. I decided one day to take it outside, put it in a bowl, and burn it page by page. I can't even tell you how good this felt. Clearing that energy away and no longer having the burden of having it beside my bed was the best thing I could have done. Of course I'll always have my memories, and that's okay. I wouldn't want to forget my past, because that's what has taught me the most. But I can do without the physical representation and constant reminder of my less-than-happy moments.

For years I held on to pieces of my show wardrobe from dancing on tour with Janet Jackson. While being on that tour was the best time of my life, it was also a very hard time for me emotionally. There was a lot going on then. I was young and naïve and didn't always make the best decisions. Now, don't get me wrong, touring with Janet will always be one of the best memories of my life. Getting to see the world, performing in stadiums and arenas filled with screaming fans, having sleepover parties with Janet and her dancers—this was all a dream come true for me. But I was young, younger than everyone else on the tour by at least six years, and had a deep desire for people to like me. I was always looked at as and treated like the baby of the group. I didn't get invited to go out as much as everyone else at night because they'd have to sneak me in with a fake ID. I wasn't asked to go to dinners because they all thought they would somehow corrupt me, the baby. Not wanting to be left out, I spent a lot of my time trying to fit in, hoping the dancers and Janet would think I was "cool." Ultimately, I was not being myself. I wanted the boys to have crushes on me. I wanted the girls to be my friends. I was nineteen and twenty years old, fighting so hard to figure out who I was. Sometimes I look back or see pictures of myself out late at clubs or trying to pretend to play poker with the other dancers and I just want to hug my former self and say, "Be yourself—everything will work out!"

So whenever I would come across the show paraphernalia it would remind me of my naïveté, taking me back to a time in my life that makes me cringe at my behavior. I got to a point where I knew I couldn't continue jabbing at my spirit every time I came across a pair of shoes or pants, regardless of where they came from. So I decided it was time to give them away. Someone else would connect an entirely different emotion to these articles. To them, they'd represent excitement and beauty and, hello, JANET. I surprisingly had no guilt giving these things away. It was as if I had risen above the memories from my past.

We often hold on to stuff (there's that word again!) because we're afraid that by giving something away, we'll lose something, but I've found the opposite. It ultimately feels better to release it and move forward. Now, on the flip side, I'll never let go of my Janet tour jacket; seeing that always makes me feel a sense of accomplishment and pride. Sometimes there's no rhyme or reason as to why a particular item makes us feel a certain way. I choose not to question but rather listen to my heart. And my heart loves that jacket.

SACRED SPACE

I feel it is important for every person, whether you live alone, with roommates, or a partner, have kids or not, to have their own sacred space that is meant only for them. When you have kids, nothing seems to be your own anymore. There is one spot in my house that is off-limits to everyone but me. Evie respects this space because she sees that I respect the space. Some people have a whole room, others a corner or even just a special chair. I have a small area in my bedroom by the window

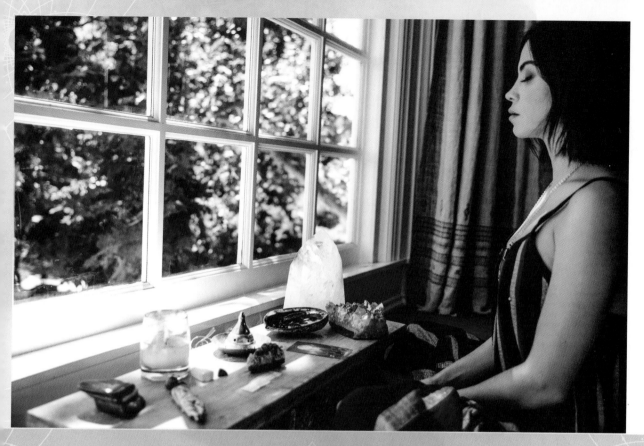

I try to create as many moments
of sacred space as possible.

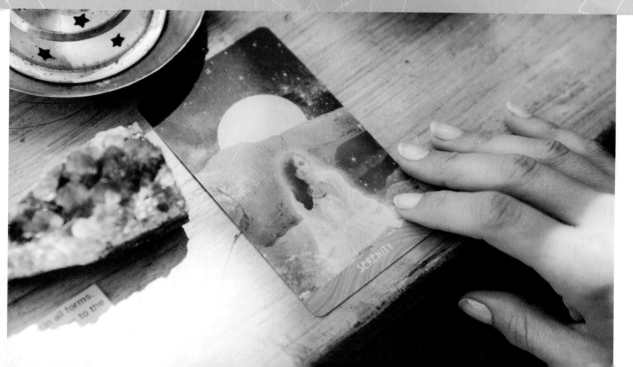

where I keep a small, low table—some might call it an altar—and a fold-up meditation chair I got on Amazon for under fifty dollars. I use this space daily as a place to set my intentions, meditate, say a mantra, or pull an angel card. I also create this space and time for myself to manifest New Year's wishes (I prefer the word *wishes* to *resolutions*). I go here to make vision boards, daydream and imagine.

Others might use this area to pray, reflect, or take ten minutes to listen to their breath. I do these things, too. Whatever your purpose or need, sacred space is not only a great reminder to keep up these rituals but also a special place to practice them. Having a designated spot is much more significant than saying, *Oh, I'll have this moment to myself in bed or at my desk,* because there's something intentional about going to a space purposed to accommodate these breaks. For me, seeing my meditation chair is also a great reminder to fit it in if I haven't yet that day.

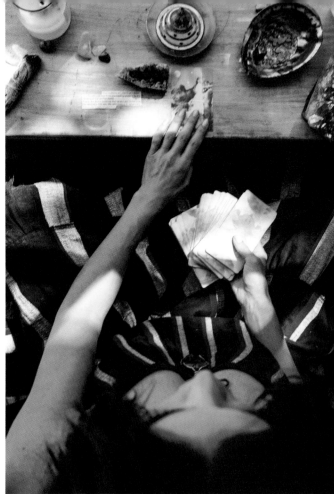

I try to create as many moments of sacred space as possible. In fact, I'm writing this from my hotel room right now, where next to the bed on a table I have my crystals, palo santo (smudge sticks), and oracle cards. I make it a point to bring these things along to provide me with a sense of home wherever I go, whether it's an on-set trailer in Hollywood or a hotel suite halfway across the world.

When I was pregnant with Evie, Channing and I were living in London, where he was filming the movie *Jupiter Ascending*. From five months into my pregnancy we lived here, away from our friends and family. Since Chan was working every day, I was for the most part on my own. I happened to be very okay with this, because as an only child who moved around every few years, I am used to acclimating to new places and making myself comfortable.

Still, I was craving a ritual in London, something to make me feel grounded and connected to something. I began the routine of getting up for a hike every day through Hampstead Heath park. If you're not familiar with it, this area is very enchanting. It has these massive fairy-tale trees with outstretched, beautiful roots. One day I was hiking through the wooded park when I made my way off the beaten path only to discover this magical-looking tree. This tree became the sacred space I would visit every day. It made me feel at peace and at home. I'd sit against its trunk to feel the heaviness of the roots and the

weight of the tree. Connecting to something so solid and stable made me feel strong when I needed it most. When I returned years later, it felt as if I was coming home. This tree feels so deeply personal to me because I made it part of my ritual and it became my sacred place. Spending time there in the past offered a special moment when I would connect to Evie in my belly, to nature, and to myself.

Having this cherished spot in London inspired me to have an outdoor one at home. We have an oak tree in my backyard, which has really become both Evie's and my special place. She has decorated it with things that are meaningful to her—for example, a small door she believes fairies come in and out of. For this reason, we call it the Fairy Tree. Sometimes I encourage the sense of magic by leaving little gifts or notes from the fairies by the tree for her to find. The you-picked-up-your-room fairy and the good-day-at-school fairy have made quite a few appearances!

I also keep a few gifts by the Fairy Tree from one of my best friends who passed

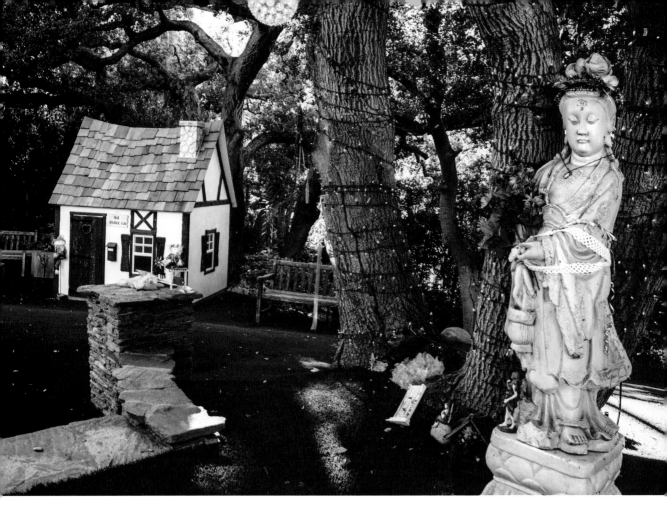

away. At the time she gave them to me she was facing a terminal diagnosis. I learned so much from her. She was not only one of my best friends, but also a life coach and healer. One of the gifts she gave me is a very personal crystal and the other, a statue of Kuan Yin, the goddess of compassion, love, and openhearted-ness. When I sit beside this statue I am reminded to connect with my friend and

all of life. I think of all the blessings of life my friend brought to me, and it brings me a real sense of peace. I find when you have something tangible to look at, something to touch, it's far more significant than a memory living in your mind. Every time I walk by the Fairy Tree I think of her, and whenever I take a moment to connect at the Fairy Tree, I feel our bond.

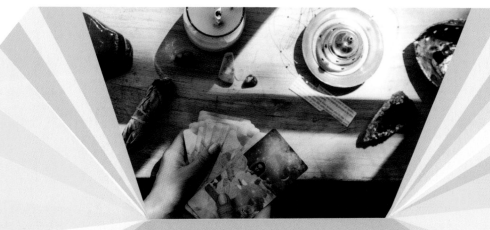

my table or altar must-haves

CANDLES. Candles are very important to me. I always have a white candle, because to me it represents purity and cleansing. You can set any intention before a white candle. If a different color speaks to you, go with that. Different scents and colors speak to us in various ways. I set my intention as I light the candle. I believe the flame activates that intention, setting it off into the world.

JOURNAL AND PEN. This is the perfect time to reflect and record it all.

VISUAL MANIFESTATION. A photo or written quote to support and inspire you.

OBJECT. Something tangible to hold and connect to. It can be a crystal or a sentimental token.

INSPIRATIONAL BEING. Some people might have a statue or image of a god or goddess. I have a little Buddha.

ANGEL OR ORACLE CARDS. These bring me a sense of connection and peace.

Someone very special to me once gave me a single die he found on the street. It lives on my altar, in my sacred space. The die became important to us both, reminding us to "roll the dice" and take chances.

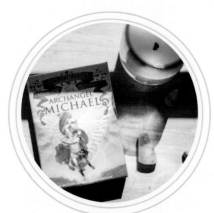

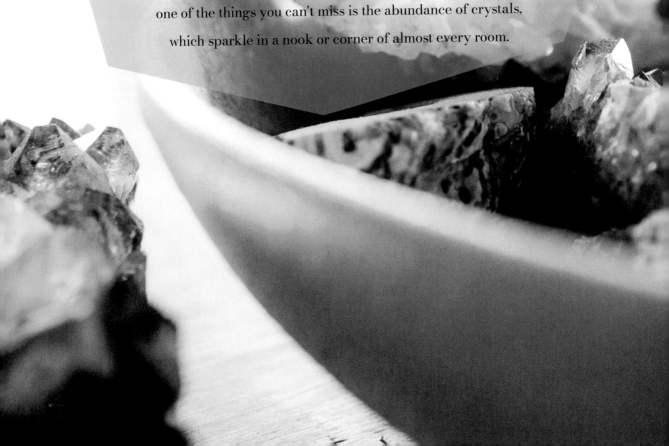

CRYSTALS

Everything and everyone is composed of energy, and the vibration created by that energy varies in quality and abundance. A higher vibration is connected to light, positivity, love, and peace. A lower vibration is connected to darkness, anxiety, fear, and sadness. Both live inside all of us. Life isn't about denying your shadow side; it's about embracing it all while choosing to give more of your attention to higher thoughts. I believe that the higher your vibration, the more likely you are to succeed in your intentions and live a gratifying life. There are many things you can do to raise your vibration, and one of them is to fill your home with high-vibrational crystals. I believe in making your space feel as lovely and positive as possible (whatever that looks like to you!). When you walk around my house, one of the things you can't miss is the abundance of crystals, which sparkle in a nook or corner of almost every room.

Crystals carry a natural energy that many (including myself, obviously) believe have healing capabilities, which benefit us by working with our own personal vibrations in various ways. They, in return, can benefit from our energy as well. Not to be confused with rocks, crystals are made of active material. They're alive! I've sought out crystals for protection, grounding, heart healing, and mental and spiritual growth. At home, crystals are my way of balancing energy and setting the tone for a more harmonious environment.

I first started collecting crystals when I moved to LA after touring with Janet. I was at the beginning of my spiritual quest and by happenstance wandering through a mall when I came across a kiosk selling crystals. Immediately I was very taken by the display. Every piece sparkled in its own way, and there was a stunning array of colors. I considered purchasing a few, thinking they'd be really pretty to have in my apartment. When the girl working the kiosk explained that crystals have actual meaning, purpose, and a reason, it changed everything. It was the first time I'd even heard the word *vibration* used in a spiritual context. From there, a whole new world opened up to me—one that was not only magical but useful, too.

My first crystal was a rose quartz, the stone of the heart. It carries feminine energy of love, peace, and nourishment. I kept the rose quartz with me always. It was either by my bed, in my bra, or around my neck. I manifested everything I wanted to bring into my life through that crystal. And I believe it worked. I still travel everywhere with a crystal. They go everywhere I go. Lately I've been carrying with me a small labradorite, stone of transformation. This iridescent blue, turquoise, and green crystal is one of the most beautiful, I think. I've been going through a lot of changes in my life, including becoming a single woman and mother. Labradorite is known to inspire strength, perseverance, and self-discovery. It is also known for its intuition-promoting abilities. It's one of my favorite crystals to give as a gift. I have a small one I've been carrying with me all the time. I'll take all the help I can get.

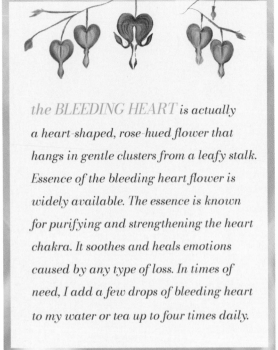

the BLEEDING HEART is actually a heart-shaped, rose-hued flower that hangs in gentle clusters from a leafy stalk. Essence of the bleeding heart flower is widely available. The essence is known for purifying and strengthening the heart chakra. It soothes and heals emotions caused by any type of loss. In times of need, I add a few drops of bleeding heart to my water or tea up to four times daily.

Especially in Western culture, we believe more is better. Can't sleep? Take this prescription and knock yourself out. Feeling blue? Your doctor can get you some pills that make feelings a thing of the past. Of course there are mental health situations when medication is essential; however, on a smaller scale, when it comes to situational anxiety, fear, sadness, and so on, I've found gentle approaches can be really powerful. Sometimes you might think you need something stronger, heavier, and more hard-core when truly a

piece of rose quartz and essence of bleeding heart will help you just as much.

When I was twenty-three I went through an extremely painful breakup. For two years, we were back and forth, on and off, as I was being pulled to and fro by this guy. The moment I finally declared I was done with my part in the relationship, things between us got very contentious and unkind. I was feeling sad, doubting myself, and just plain heartbroken. One of my friends introduced me to a bleeding heart remedy, which I took a couple of times a day. I also started wearing an aquamarine crystal, which symbolizes strength, happiness, and healing. Within weeks it was as if the dawn started to break. I noticed colors differently, smiled more, felt hopeful overall. I was over my ordeal and ready to move onward, forward. It was a great lesson for me to feel firsthand the power of connecting to the earth and the subtler approaches to healing with the inner rhythm of life.

My most treasured crystal is a rare one: a Brazilian grandfather quartz. My friend

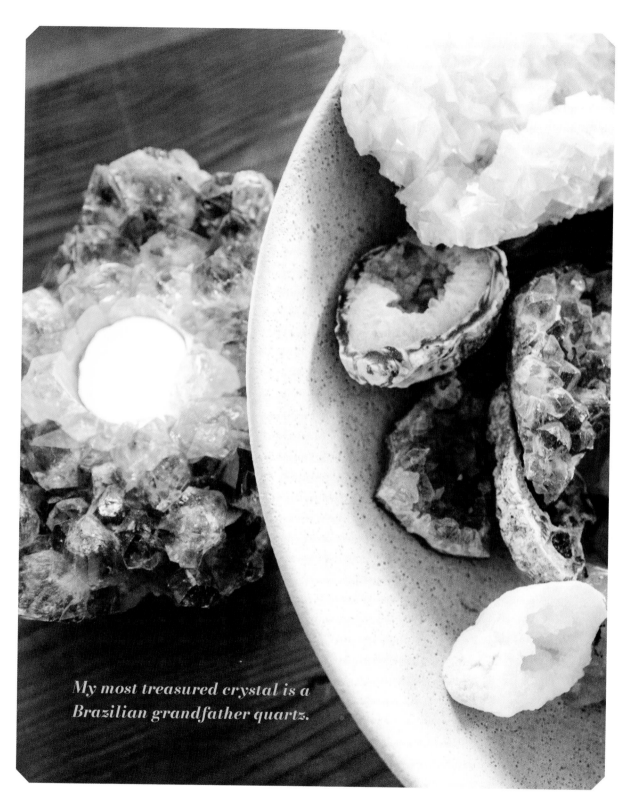

*My most treasured crystal is a
Brazilian grandfather quartz.*

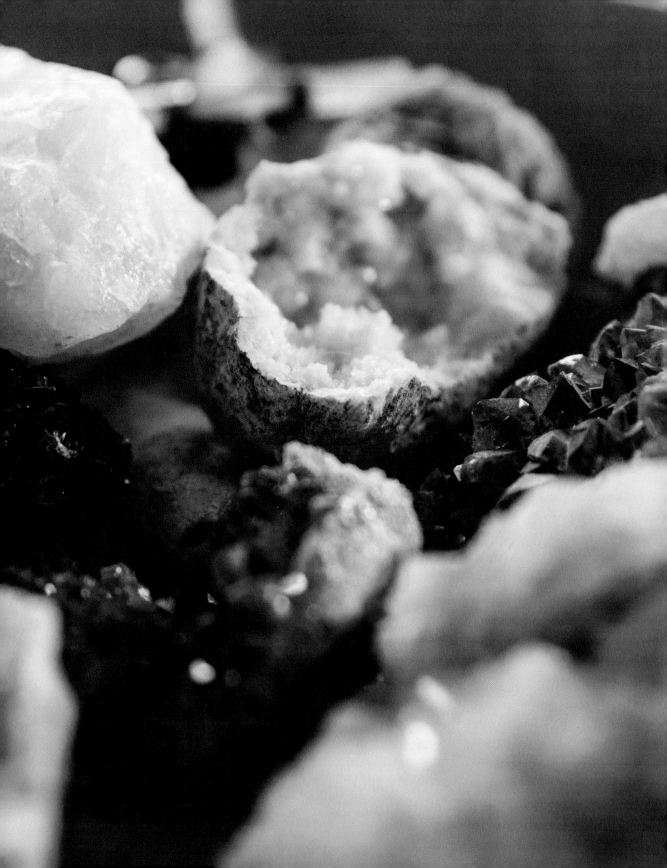

Nicole found it years ago at a flea market. It was beaten up, broken, and barren looking, but Nicole saw past its flaws and took it home. My friend put it in her sacred space, where she gave it love and positive energy over the years. I kid you not, the crystals slowly but surely started to repair and look better overall. I watched this crystal go from bleak to beautiful. I saw it with my own eyes. We forget that crystals are from the earth and that they carry energy. Like a plant or anything else containing life, they can heal and grow. I was honored when Nicole gifted me this crystal. It now lives in my sacred space under the Fairy Tree. Every time I walk by it I think of her. I love it.

The best thing about crystals is that they kind of find you. I personally don't like to buy crystals online. I enjoy the process of going to a store with an open mind and waiting to see what speaks to me. I'll hold each crystal, read about its properties, and let my spirit guide me toward a connection. In a funny way it's not much different from adopting a puppy or kitten, where you'd seek out a mutual bond rather than pick a pet based on looks alone.

my favorite HIGH-VIBRATION CRYSTALS

ROSE QUARTZ. *For your heart chakra.* Carry one on you or place it near you: in your pocket, by your bed, in your car, wherever makes you happy.

SMOKY QUARTZ. *This is for protection and grounding.* Excellent to have by your bed at dreamtime; you will never see me traveling without one in my pocket.

HEMATITE. *Another excellent crystal for grounding.* For big meetings and overwhelming situations, always carry some hematite.

AMETHYST. *Calming, opens intuition and your third-eye chakra.* I sometimes lie down and hold this crystal during a nap or place it under my pillow. This is overall vibration increasing and intuition opening.

CLEAR QUARTZ. *Like the white candle, clear quartz can be programmed with any intention you desire!* Incredible for cleaning the aura and bringing clarity of mind.

LABRADORITE. *Visionary, expansive, the seer stone.* This is a protective and magical crystal that can open up your intuition. My favorite one! I have one I carry with me and a large one in my bedroom as well.

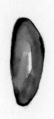

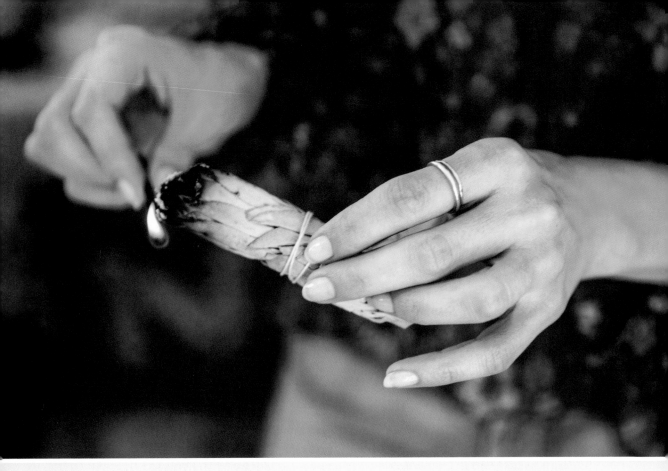

SAGE ADVICE

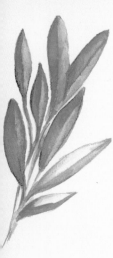

- ▲ **WHITE SAGE** *is considered a sacred, powerful plant. It can be dried, bound into a bunch, and burned. The smoke this produces gathers negativity, leaving only positivity behind. Commonly used in the home, over people, and on objects.*

- ▲ **PALO SANTO** *in Spanish translates to "holy wood." The dense piece of wood is known for being a powerful energetic cleanser with medicinal healing properties.*

- ▲ **COPAL** *is made of tree resin and looks like a stick of incense. It's meant to cleanse spaces and objects with its clean, light, woody scent. In Peru, you'll walk into a restaurant to find they have this burning all the time.*

When it comes to energetic cleansing, my go-to tools of choice are white sage, palo santo, and copal. There was a time when I tried to clear my house with tobacco, which I learned from a shaman in Peru. Tobacco is a very powerful plant, although it smells exactly how you think it does. Another time I tried an out-there remedy involving Epsom salt, Everclear, and fire. Let's just say I've since stuck to burning herbs and wood to shift the energy around in my house!

For me, space clearing is a staple practice. So often it feels like we could use new energy or a new beginning, especially following an argument or unfortunate event. I think of it almost like sweeping the dust off your shelves or mopping the floors. The air smells better, fresher, and your mind is even more right knowing your space is clean and new. Clearing the air is bigger than that, as it offers a new beginning where you can create space for fresh energy to enter and allow you to start anew.

I've had to explain this process to a few people in my life, namely some very concerned firemen. One day I was going pretty hard-core on the copal when suddenly the fire alarms started going off. I threw the sticks in the sink and started wafting smoke through every window I could get to in my strongest effort to clear the air. Before I knew it, there were fire trucks, sirens, lights and all. "I'm so sorry, I was saging the house and . . ." I tried to explain. "You mean burning incense?" I could see their eyes rolling all around me. I was probably the third hippie lady with a false fire alarm that week.

But . . . it really does work for me! I think you'll love the difference in the air. Just don't forget to open the windows.

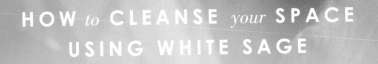

HOW *to* CLEANSE *your* SPACE
USING WHITE SAGE

Sage smudging is the most common practice
to release and clear energy.

1. Light one end of the bundle of herbs with a match, lighter, or candle.

2. Set an intention for the sage. What are you clearing out and what do you
wish to invite in?

3. Move around the space with the above intentions in mind as you direct the
smoke into the areas in need of clearing. I like to direct smoke into the corners of each room and over areas or objects in need of special attention.

4. Observe the smoke and all the negativity it carries as it exits through an
open window or door to the outside.

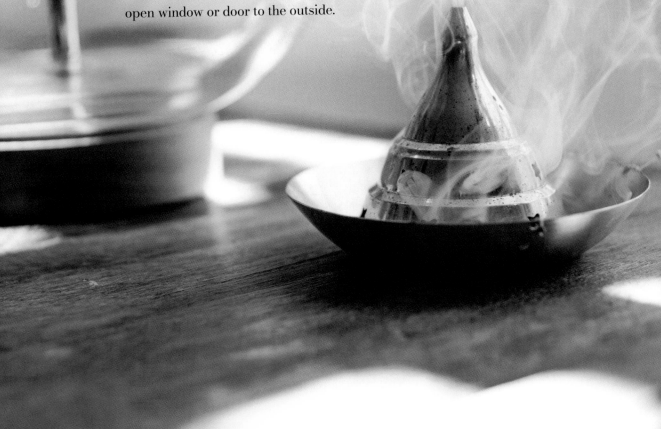

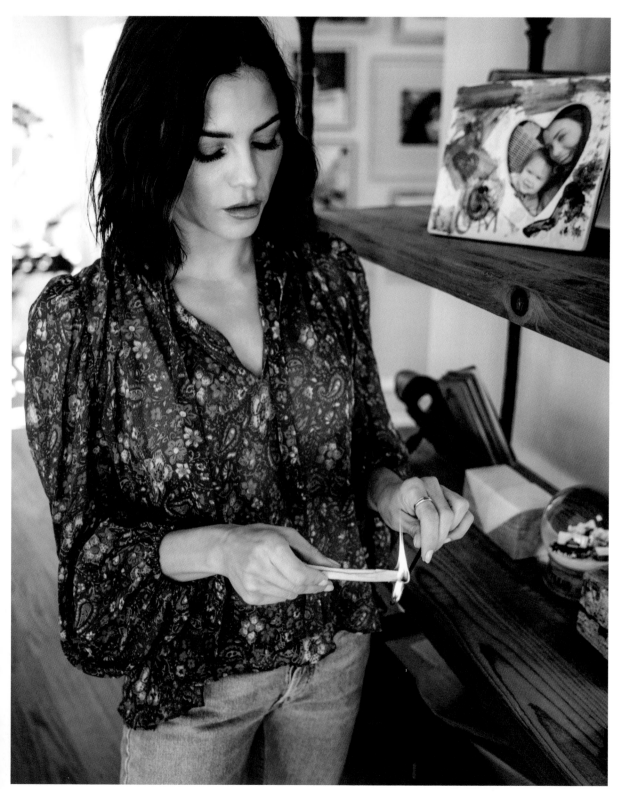

FLOWER WATER

Essential oils play a huge role in my life. I always rub a few drops of clary sage on my belly before a menstrual cycle, diluted peppermint on the bottoms of Evie's and my feet to bring a fever down, and I'm constantly filling a room with feel-good oils from my Young Living oil diffuser.

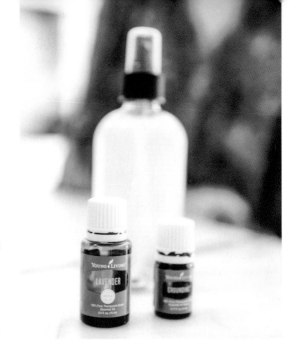

Another way I like to work with aromatherapy is by using what I call flower water. Although if you ask my daughter, it's called "Evie's Bug Spray," because for some reason she believes it's to keep creepy crawlers out of her room. Little does she know her bug spray is actually calming her down at bedtime. She always asks, "Did you spray the bug spray?" I use this spray to encourage peace and serenity in the house. It's a gentle space and energy healer that smells divine.

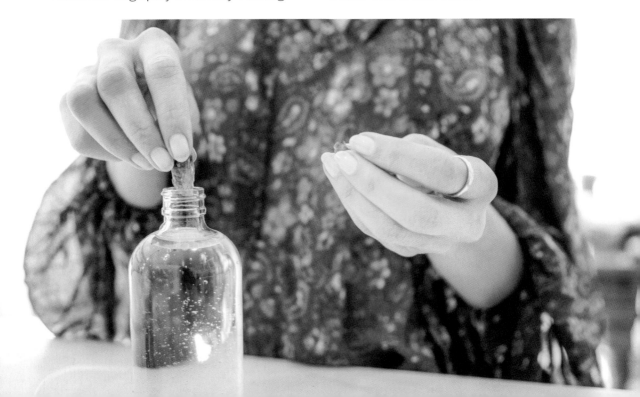

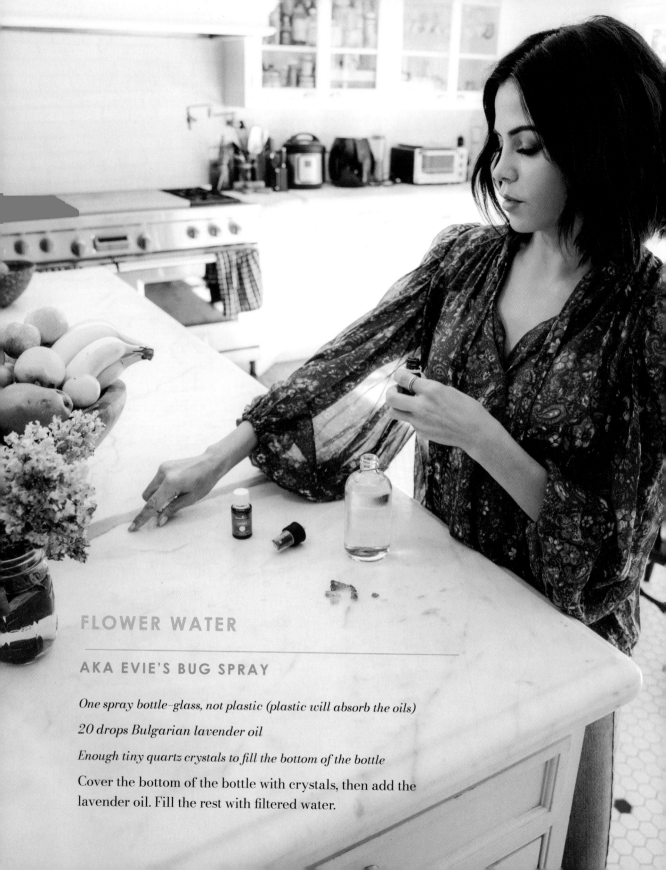

FLOWER WATER

AKA EVIE'S BUG SPRAY

One spray bottle–glass, not plastic (plastic will absorb the oils)

20 drops Bulgarian lavender oil

Enough tiny quartz crystals to fill the bottom of the bottle

Cover the bottom of the bottle with crystals, then add the
lavender oil. Fill the rest with filtered water.

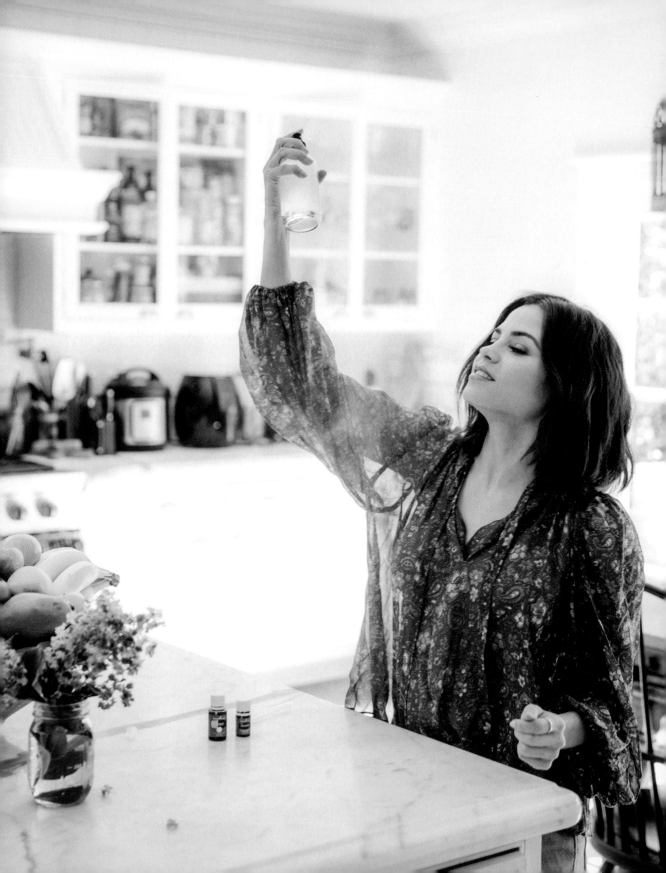

TAKE WITH YOU

If you look at your home as a reflection of who
you want to be or how you want to feel, it greatly
changes how you go about nurturing your space.
Something as simple as organizing a junk drawer
can make a huge difference in the chaos you might
be experiencing emotionally. I agree with the
sentiment "A cluttered home equates to a cluttered
mind." You spend your most intimate moments
in this space. It should support you emotionally,
physically, and spiritually. Whether you do a full-on
Marie Kondo purging of the whole house or spend
a short amount of time saging a room after an
argument, every intentional choice to clear your
home will only elevate how you feel in it.

if there is grace

in your heart,

in your bones,

in your breath,

you will always be beautiful.

—APRIL GREEN

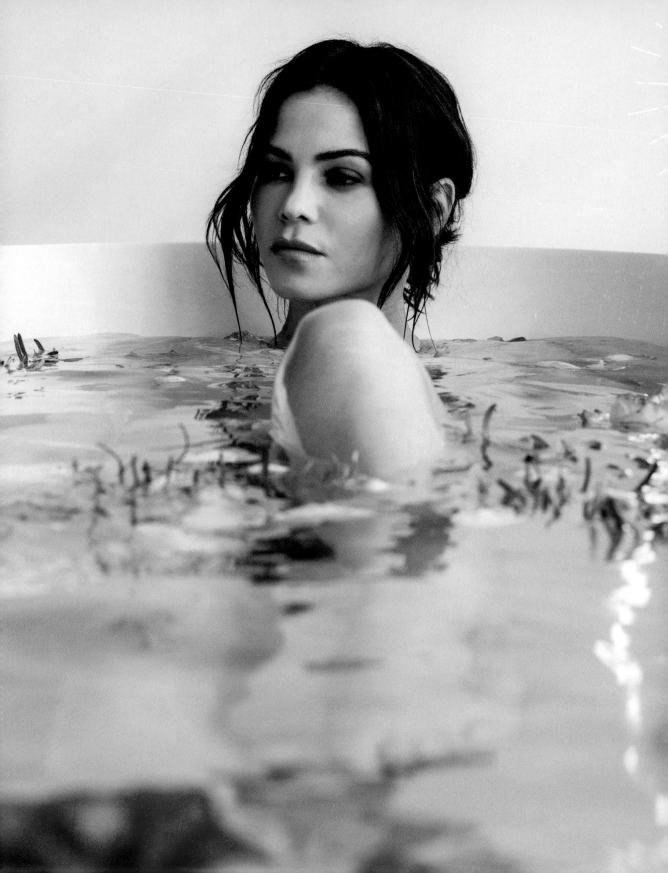

CHAPTER THREE

---

inner beauty rituals

wholeheartedly believe our inner beauty directly affects our outer beauty. When we feel beautiful on the inside, we in turn act, feel, and present ourselves more beautifully. You might spend an hour primping, but you won't be able to truly hide your discontent from the world if you're feeling badly. There isn't a contour kit out there to make you believe you look like a beauty queen when you're harboring sadness, stress, or disappointment. Or, if you're an empath like me, when you're holding on to somebody else's unfortunate situation. I've had days when I was stewing over something, either an unresolved argument or an impending decision. Meanwhile, my glam squad would deck me out from head to toe for a photo shoot. Even with all their magic, I wasn't able to see what everyone else said they saw when I looked into the mirror, because all I recognized was the anxiety hiding behind my eyes. I wasn't capable of feeling my best; therefore, I didn't believe I looked my best either.

Feeling discontent isn't always about what's going on in my life. Personally, I consider myself to be a hard-core empath. Some people define an empath as someone who is able to pick up on other people's thoughts almost like a clairvoyant could. I describe my empathy type more along the lines of adopting other people's feelings and energy. If I come across someone who is having the worst possible day, I don't merely sympathize by feeling badly for that person. If I'm not careful, I can actually take on their emotions as if the worst possible day is happening to

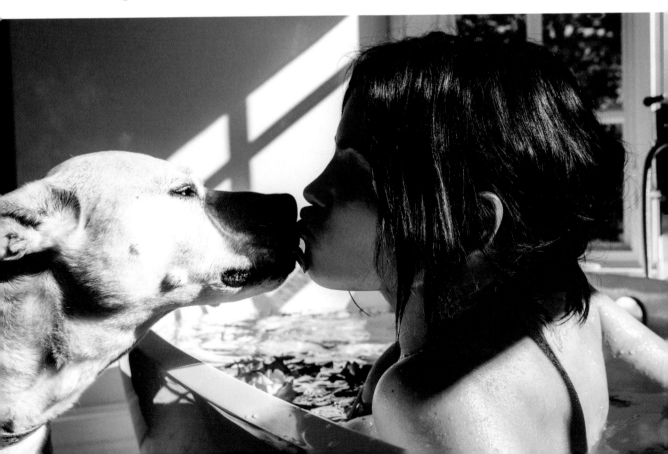

me, too. Sometimes hours after spending time with that person I might be wondering why I'm feeling a little heavy. It will take a minute before I realize, *Aha! This mess isn't mine*. But being empathetic isn't necessarily a negative thing. It has many positive attributes to it as well. For one, an empath is very compassionate in regard to other people's feelings. I'm able to tune in to others' emotions and have a very keen sense of what is happening for them, which, as a friend, helps me give great advice. But on the flip side, if you were to come over to my house, curl up on my couch, and list all your latest stresses, that anxiety wouldn't leave my home as you reversed down my driveway. I would feel these feelings with you, and your worries would stick with me, becoming my issues as well if I'm not careful.

Like anything else, I believe a healthy amount of empathy is best in moderation. Ideally, we would sympathize with someone, put ourselves in their shoes momentarily, and understand why they're upset without us ourselves feeling upset on their behalf. That would be my happy medium if I had a choice. But that's not who I am. So I've had to learn how to shield myself and create healthy boundaries. It is still a work in progress, but by learning to say no, accepting only mutually fulfilling relationships and friendships in my life, and learning to give no more than 50 percent in any relationship, I have felt much better.

Being an empath affects my inner beauty because often other people's negativity clouds my thoughts and casts a shadow over my spirit. As much as I try to shield myself from taking on other people's stories, I don't necessarily have a choice in this regard. However, there are ways to shake off whatever I've taken on throughout the day. I've found that by practicing certain rituals on a regular basis I am able to discern and free myself from whatever feelings and associations are not my own.

Besides emotion, we carry a great deal of information within us all day, every day. The stress of a tough day can sit in your gut, rest on your shoulders, or hover inside your chest. Emotions are rarely ever just "in your head." They take up residence in your whole body. Holding on to this toxicity can lead to issues like illness, fatigue, and depression, to name a few. For these reasons it is absolutely essential for us to regularly practice a type of self-care I call "spiritual hygiene." Since I do take on the worries of others in addition to my own, I feel even more of a need to release not only my own toxic energy but the negativity I take on from others, too. I think of it like this: we brush our teeth, shampoo our hair, and exfoliate our skin to remove plaque, dirt, and dead skin. It's part of our daily hygiene, what we do to stay fresh and clean. Why wouldn't we practice the same type of cleansing from the inside? Do we not need to give our emotions and our spirit a purifying scrub-down, too?

At the end of the day, I like to go to bed with clean skin, fresh breath, and a clear conscience. They all go hand in hand. Some days I have more me time to take advantage of and focus on my spiritual hygiene. Others, I'm lucky to squeeze in

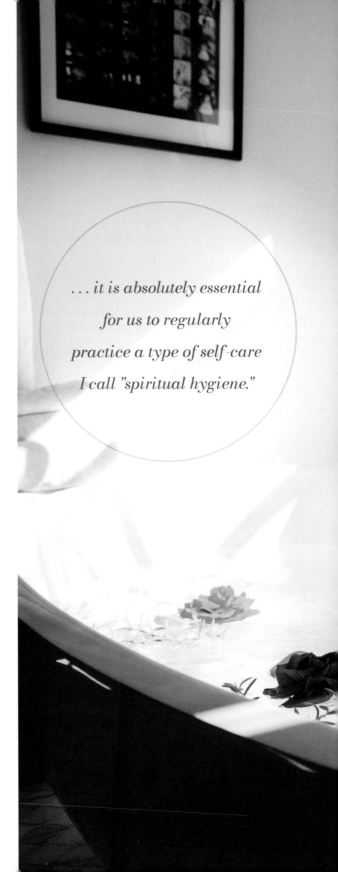

. . . it is absolutely essential for us to regularly practice a type of self-care I call "spiritual hygiene."

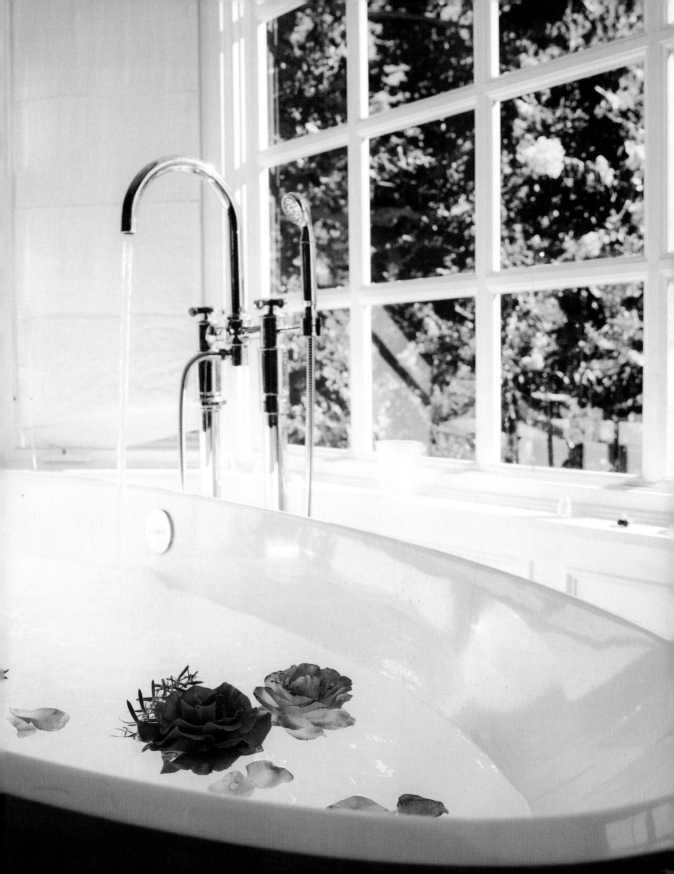

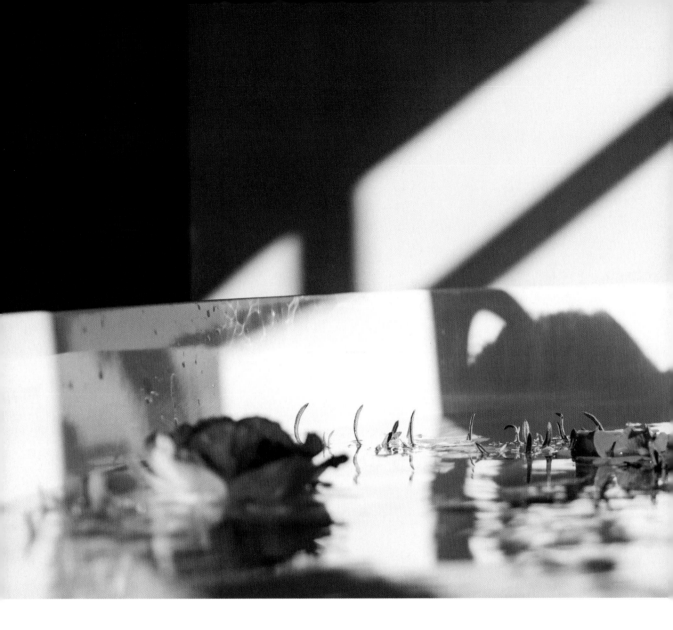

ten minutes of visualization or breath-work. Either way, it's incredibly important for me to get in what I can in order to feel internally clear and beautiful.

PLANT BATHS

Years ago, for my birthday I went by my-self to Peru for two weeks. It was a retreat from the city, meetings, and the everyday hustle that is regular life. My intention was to self-nurture, soak up the alone time,

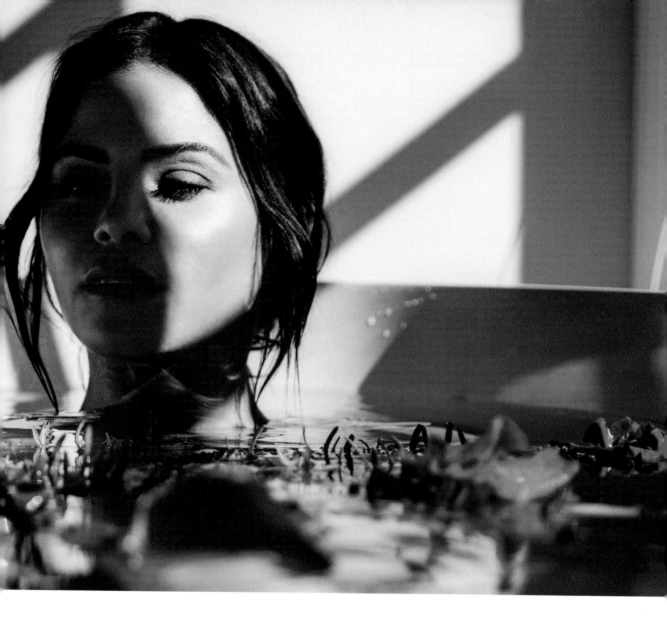

and reflect on my life with gratitude. I lived with the women of a very beautiful Amazonian tribe. One of the rituals they taught me was to take plant baths. The community of women would get together around a yurt to prepare the baths. They used local master plants such as *ajo sacha* and *piñon blanco*. *Ajo sacha* is an Amazonian power plant also known as "jungle garlic" due to its garlicky scent. The wild leafy plant features violet flowers and is said to offer us protection and break us of unwanted attachments. *Piñon blanco* might look and smell like typical ivy; however, it is believed to give strength to the energies of the body, mind, and soul. I worked alongside the women as we broke these plants down with our hands, ground them down with a mortar and pestle, and added them to a tub along with lime, sea salt, menthol, and Florida water. As the bath is created, it is charged with intentional thoughts of cleansing and peace of mind. Making these baths with the women was such a bonding moment for me, even though I didn't speak their language.

Once the bath had stood for a full day, I stepped into the warm, green water of my first plant bath and let my body melt in. It was like stepping into a bath of light. I felt amazing. I remember feeling an overwhelming sense of self-love and gratitude for discovering a deeper knowledge of myself. When I stepped out of the bath, I instantly felt reborn, grounded—happier, even. It was one of the major moments I'd been searching for since my youth, to feel connected to something bigger than

FLORIDA WATER is a store-bought blend of alcohol and essential oils. It's widely known for its cleansing properties and used as a perfume, bath base, or space cleanser. Florida water is especially popular in South America. People there love the citrusy scent because they believe it's similar to the scent you smell when you cross over to the afterlife.

myself. On the following days, I took the water back to my cabin, where I stood in the bathtub and poured it over my whole body. I also did this on my deck at night. I'd let the water stay on me for however long before showering. Working with the plants in this way, to clean your energy and yourself, was something that never left me. I incorporated it as much as possible into my baths at home. Granted, I couldn't just tear up a palm tree and place it in my tub, but now I substitute more readily available herbs, oils, salts, and scrubs for a similar experience.

I still use Florida water, which is easy to find online. I also incorporate a ton of sea salt into my own concoctions. One rule I always try to follow: no phone in the bathroom. Instead, I'll listen to music or meditate. I'll also visualize that whatever goes down the drain post-soak is taking the day along with it. Goodbye, lady who flipped me off in traffic. Adios, preschool drop-off tantrum. Everything I saw, everyone I talked to, every thought, issue, or emotion that isn't serving me well goes down the drain. It's like cutting a cord and letting go. With this practice, I always feel I'm in a better place to go to bed and tackle the next day.

My usual recipe for an at-home plant bath is pretty simple. While some might sprinkle only a modest amount of salts into their bath, I say bring on the salt. Sea salt is pure purifying magic! Salt crystals absorb negative energy on and around you, making you feel clear and clean from your aura to your toes. Equally important in my eyes is the addition of pure argan, coconut, or other conditioning oil. While extremely beneficial, salt can also be very drying.

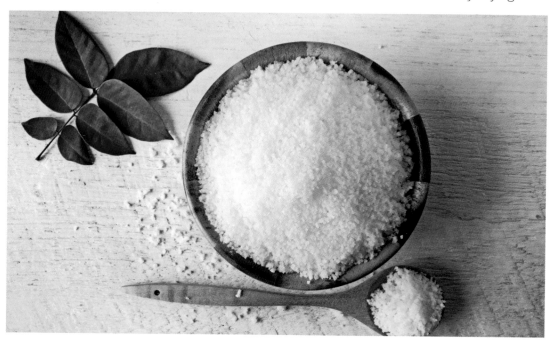

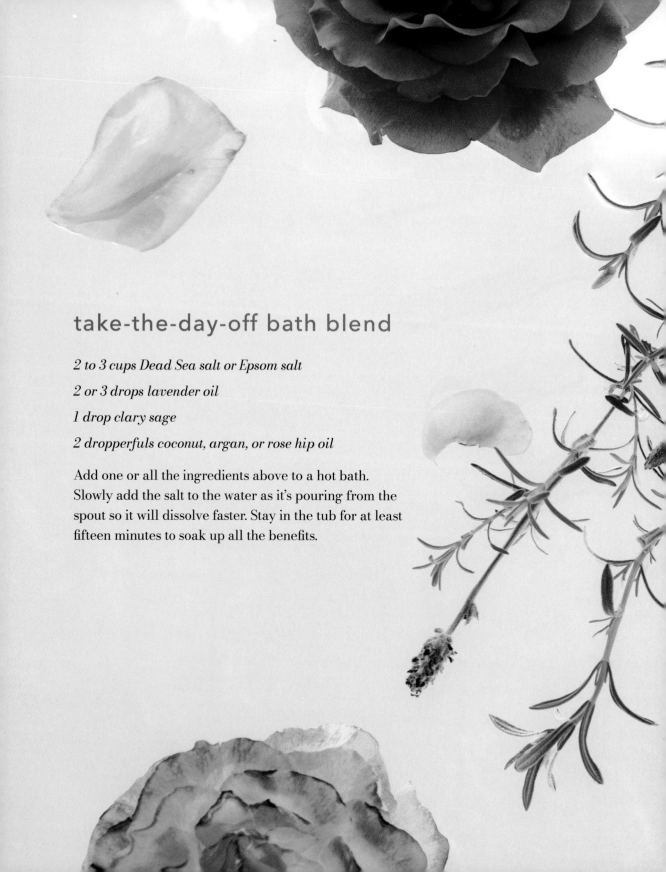

take-the-day-off bath blend

2 to 3 cups Dead Sea salt or Epsom salt

2 or 3 drops lavender oil

1 drop clary sage

2 dropperfuls coconut, argan, or rose hip oil

Add one or all the ingredients above to a hot bath.
Slowly add the salt to the water as it's pouring from the
spout so it will dissolve faster. Stay in the tub for at least
fifteen minutes to soak up all the benefits.

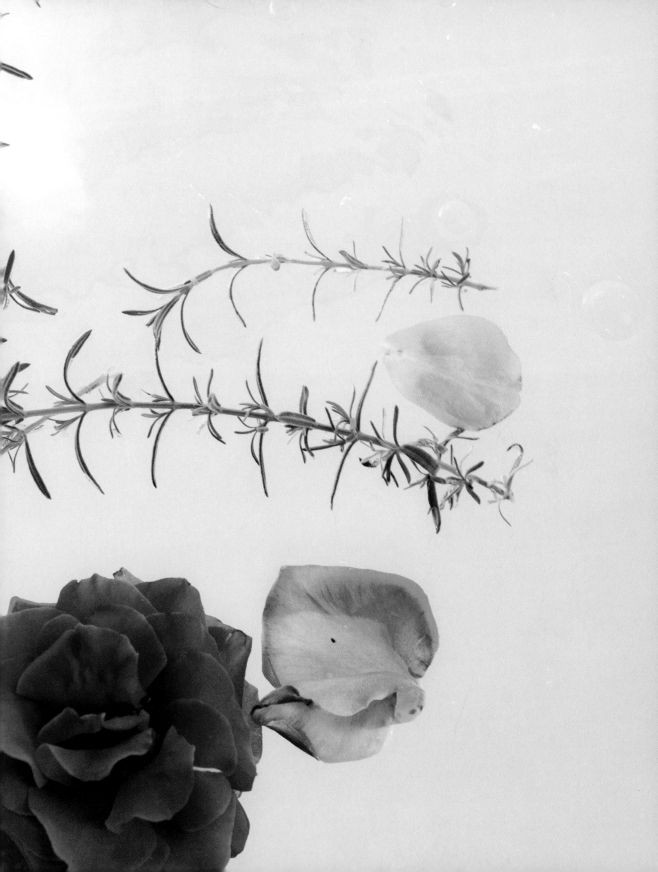

GODDESS CIRCLES

One of the most healing things a woman can do for herself is share what she's going through with another woman. I know exactly what you're thinking: *Gee thanks, Jenna. And also, the sky is blue.* Allow me to elaborate! There's a difference between calling your friend to pour your heart out when it's about to implode and setting intentional dates on a regular basis to keep each other centered and grounded. We have moms' groups, book clubs, cooking clubs, and more, but none of these get-together groups have to do with personal growth, looking within, or connecting to the divine feminine. I am a huge fan of plans where people get together to learn and grow—even if it has to do with the casserole of the week. However, my wish is for women to bond in other ways, too, ways that allow us to lift each other up and support one another on our personal journeys.

Like so many of you, I have a very busy life. I hardly get to see my friends, so when I do, I want it to be memorable and meaningful. I'm grateful to have a tribe of friends who inspire, love, and elevate each other. I believe we are not here to go about this life alone. We are meant to share it and experience it with each other. This is a huge priority for me.

One of my favorite things to do is gather my friends, especially for spiritual purposes. I've buddied up to take courses on Reiki and gone on a trip with a friend to Sedona, Arizona, where we spent the weekend scouring spiritual shops and having our auras read. While I was enjoying these fun jaunts, I began to realize they weren't bringing my friends and me closer in any real way. We were exploring and having a good time, both excellent things to do, but it was all surface level. In going on these adventures, we weren't sharing our deeply personal journeys or gaining spiritual benefits from our time away.

I'd always wanted to host some sort of get-together with like-minded women to chat and connect over our spirituality. I was very fortunate to meet a female shaman who specializes in cacao ceremonies, something I knew I wanted to do the moment I heard about it. In these gatherings, cacao is used for medicinal purposes: it's intended to cleanse your aura, to open your heart and spirit.

Everyone starts by drinking a cup of hot cacao elixir, as we set our intentions and connect to ourselves, the energy in the room, and each other. I knew it would be enlightening, encouraging, and, with the right group, fun. I called up a group of my girlfriends and set the date.

The shaman who came to my house to lead our goddess circles did not disappoint. She created a welcoming environment and set the energy for the tone of our circle by having us first go around and talk about what was happening in our lives. She encouraged us to reach a level of depth that went beyond any ordinary surface conversation. Each woman took her turn not to vent but rather to talk about some of the things she was working on or through in her life. These circles allow the space for people to truly open up and address and release anything they're holding on to. We take turns talking about major life changes, everyday happenings, or occasional hiccups. The shaman had us each speak an intention and

guided us through meditations and visualizations. Everything we did was enhanced by being in a group atmosphere. It was so much more than just hanging out with the girls, because the circle allows for a deeper communication and connection among the participants. Surface feelings are bypassed: you go right to what you are dealing with deeply. The feeling of community and support is magical. Once we started getting together for goddess circles, we knew we couldn't stop. It's become a regular ritual we try our best to make time for and always look forward to.

During these circles we drink tea or cocoa, play music, read poetry, meditate, and talk about life. Sometimes there are tears, but there's always laughter and tons of hugs. The focus of the circle can change every time we meet. It can be about anything, but at its core it's really an excuse to get women together and on each other's journeys to help them support one another. Sharing these precious moments will help you to clear your your heart chakra and overcome obstacles.

CACAO tastes a lot richer and more bitter than cocoa. It's definitely not anything like the sweet powdered instant stuff we used to have as kids!

GUIDE *to* HOSTING *a*
goddess circle

▲ **SELECT AT LEAST TWO POSITIVE, OPENHEARTED, OPEN-MINDED FRIENDS.**

▲ **FIND A GOOD TIME AND DAY TO SUPPORT A SAFE SPACE.**
This isn't the best thing to do when the kids are in need of your attention or when your roommate is hosting a Super Bowl party.

▲ **SETUP** *should be in a comfortable, open, and cozy room. Supply cushions for everyone to sit on, or ask each guest to bring a yoga mat or pillow.*

▲ **CIRCLES** *make everyone feel united, so it's important for participants to maintain one.*

▲ *Create* **AMBIANCE** *with soft, gently scented candles and calm, soothing music.*

▲ **HAVE ENOUGH TEA** *ready for everyone. Sipping tea is like accepting an internal hug, and that helps everyone feel at ease.*

▲ *One of my favorite ways to initiate conversation is to have each person draw an* **ANGEL OR ORACLE CARD** *in the center of the circle. The cards will help them decide what to discuss when it's their turn to talk.*

▲ **DECIDE WHO SHOULD LEAD** *the conversation, whether it's you or a guest.*

▲ *As the host, encourage everyone to* **OPEN UP BY DIGGING A LITTLE DEEPER** *than asking, "How is work?" or "How was your day?" If someone seems stuck, try asking why they feel a certain way until they get into a productive groove.*

▲ **ENCOURAGE EVERYONE TO KEEP IT ELEVATED.** *The conversation should be about inner growth and personal journeys. It's not about ripping on our significant other or complaining about a coworker. What is going on in your life? What are you working toward? What do you want to attract to your life?*

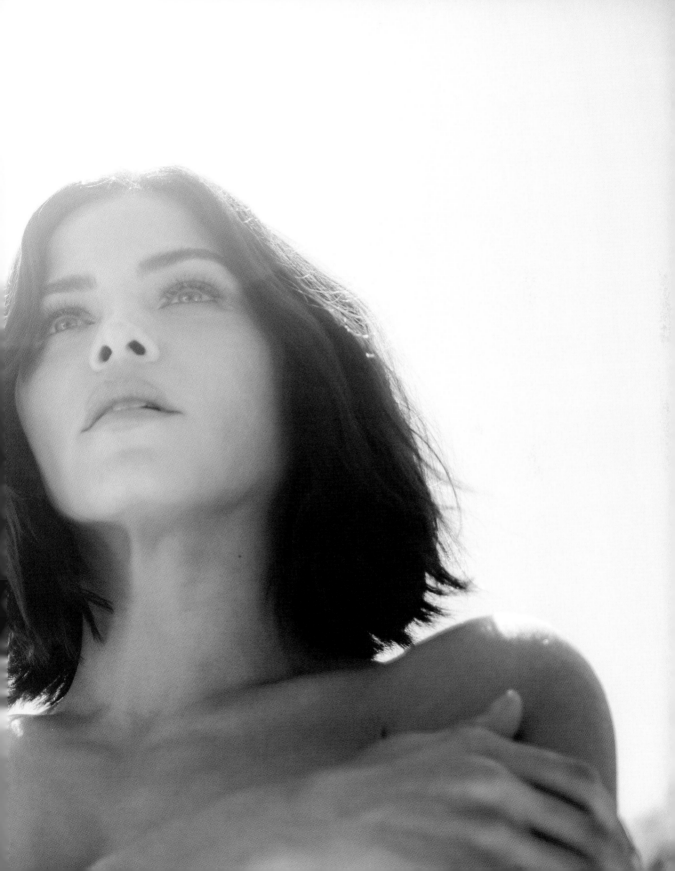

BREATHWORK

I like breathwork because it's so simple. The very first thing we do when we're born is take a breath. The very second something works out, we instinctively exhale a sigh of relief. When we get anxious or scared, we immediately hold our breath. Breathing is the essence of life. It is literally what keeps us alive, but also, it's one of the most powerful tools we have when it comes to affecting our minds and bodies. If you can remember occasionally throughout the day to let out a long, purposeful breath, you'll see how immediately potent it can be.

When I was a guest on *American Horror Story*, my character had a scene where she was high on adrenaline and fear. In order to prepare, right before we'd shoot I would give myself an intense adrenaline rush just by breathing really fast and shallowly. At the end of the day, I was absolutely exhausted. For my scenes, I didn't have to run or climb any obstacles, yet I was physically and emotionally wiped out. I remember thinking, *Wow, this is all from my breath.*

Breathwork helped me through a transition when I was at a crossroads in my life. I was confused about where I was headed and what I wanted for myself. I went to see a specialist in Holotropic Breathwork in hopes that she would help me release my fearful grip on having to know the answers. My goal was to be more go-with-the-flow, less afraid about what was ahead for me. Holotropic Breathwork is a specific practice involving intense breathing, which allows access to your deepest levels of consciousness. I had read and heard that this practice was so powerful it could alter my state of consciousness, almost like a psychedelic. I was nervous to give it a try, but I figured, how mind-altering could it be? After all, it was just breathing. I had no idea.

The practitioner had me lie on a table. She gave me grounding rocks for each hand. Then she put on a playlist and told me to breathe. She breathed along with me. She guided me into a three-point breath, where you breathe only from your mouth for two breaths in and one out. Breathing exclusively through your mouth isn't as easy as it sounds. You want to breathe through your nose by instinct. It takes concentration. That's why it's called breath*work*, I guess.

As a control freak, I wanted to stop to ask her what would happen next. I don't like letting my body go or allowing someone else to guide it. While I can go with the flow in life, it isn't the same when it comes to my physical being. Being a dancer, I've spent twenty-plus years controlling my body, so it's very hard for me to let that control go. Immediately I decided I didn't like this. I began to get light-headed and dizzy. Fearful I might pass out, I expressed concern to the facilitator, who convinced me to keep going. By the time the second song on her playlist began, I felt I might have a panic attack or fall off the bed. I was scared. She calmed me with inspirational sayings, encouraging me to let go and surrender, told me to trust my body and stick with it. Tears were streaming down my face as I encountered some internal pain I had been holding on

to. In that moment, I decided to embrace it rather than run from it. Suddenly I was flooded with a euphoric, peaceful feeling. I knew I was experiencing a breakthrough. The part of me that wanted to give up pushed through, and eventually I got myself to this blissful state of mind. I began slowly breathing through my nose as I came back to my centered self. When my session was over, I looked in the mirror and, I kid you not, my eyes were brighter; I looked lighter. "That's just the beginning," she told me. I still go back to this practice whenever I need to work through something emotionally difficult, just as I would a therapist.

On my own, I practice a different type of breathwork all the time. If I'm in a place of fight or flight, or I'm just feeling a little off, I'll put on a calm song and breathe through the entirety of that song with deep belly breaths. On the inhale through my nose I'll take in a deep breath all the way until it fills my belly and then slowly exhale through my mouth.

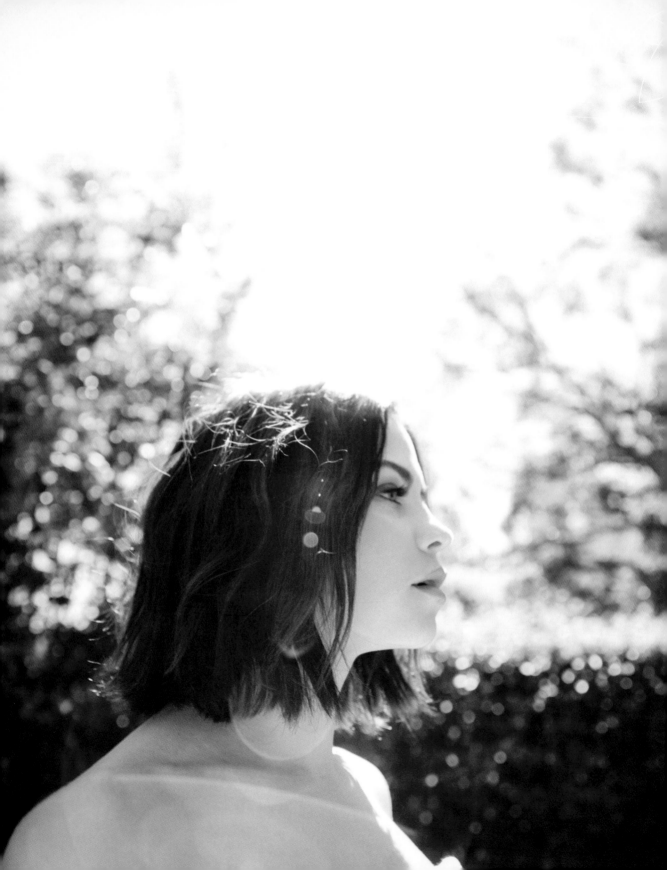

4-7-8 BREATHWORK

The 4-7-8 breathing technique was developed by
Dr. Andrew Weil. This particular pattern of breathing benefits
us in a multitude of ways. By focusing on our breath, we pay
less attention to our worries, stressors, and anxieties. As we
deliver delicious oxygen to our organs and tissues, our minds
are set at ease. I practice the 4-7-8 when I'm really working
through something, or even just when I'm in need of an
excellent night's sleep.

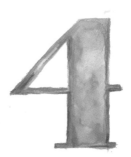

▲ GET COMFORTABLE.

▲ WITH RELAXED LIPS, LOUDLY EXHALE COMPLETELY
THROUGH YOUR MOUTH.

▲ CLOSE YOUR LIPS AND INHALE SILENTLY THROUGH
YOUR NOSE AS YOU COUNT TO FOUR IN YOUR
HEAD.

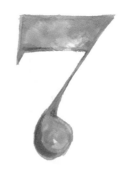

▲ HOLD YOUR BREATH FOR SEVEN SECONDS.

▲ AUDIBLY EXHALE THROUGH YOUR MOUTH
FOR EIGHT SECONDS.

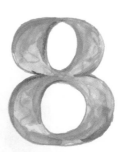

   When you're first starting out, it is recommended you do
this for only four breaths. With practice, gradually work your
way up to eight full breaths.

VISUALIZATION

A few years ago, I was in a place of wanting to feel a little more fulfilled by the work I was doing. While I was appreciative of having work to do, I just didn't feel like I was doing what I was meant to. Oprah defines authentic power as when you use your gifts, talents, and personality to serve the purpose of your soul. I felt I wasn't using any of these things, and therefore I felt very lost. It was as if I was wandering through life waiting for an opportunity to show up, something that would look the way I had always thought the perfect opportunity would look. I switched it up and began to practice a visualization where I would make myself feel how I would if I was working on a project that made me feel fulfilled. For me this conjured up feelings of excitement and confidence. I knew it would involve engaging and connecting with other people while having fun. It should be fun, right?! I imagined myself feeling lighthearted and free to express my authentic self. I didn't know if these feelings would come from a television show or a movie, but I truly didn't care. I surrendered to the unknown outcome.

A couple of months down the line my agent called to discuss a new show called *World of Dance*. I wasn't sure how I felt about hosting a competition show. At the time, I was actually developing a different dance show. With an open mind, I visualized what it would feel like to host *World of Dance*. Lo and behold, it was the same feeling I was seeking out. It felt GOOD. I'd connect with other dancers, get to be my true self, be around music I loved, get to dance a bit, and be around the fun energy I was hoping for. It was a major "aha" moment for me. This was what I'd manifested. It wasn't the opportunity I'd thought it was going to be, but it ended up being extremely fulfilling and fun. It was exactly what I needed at the time. I believe that had I not worked on my visualizations and not known what elements I was looking for, I wouldn't have seen this great opportunity for all that it was.

Visualizations constantly come into play. To be honest, I pretty much do them all day long, all the time. Below are my favorite ways to work with visualizations. Give them a try!

imagination visualization

Even though I've been performing all my life, I still get nervous from time to time. You never know how a talk show appearance is going to pan out or whether an audition is going to go in your favor. The same goes for first dates, interviews, even walking down the aisle, or going into any exciting life event. What I like to do at least five minutes beforehand is take the time to imagine what it would look and feel like if everything went as well as could be expected. I visualize every step, every moment, successfully happening in real time, allowing myself to experience lit-up emotions. Doing so always calms my nerves, sets the tone for my confidence, and grounds me for what is to come.

energy barrier visualization

You know those crazy wind tunnel tubes people used to stand in as they tried to grab money on television game shows? Sometimes I imagine something similar, but for me, it's a wind tunnel filled with white light. If I'm sitting in my car or on set in a trailer, I'll visualize this feeling of white light racing up from my feet, climbing up my back in a circular motion. It speeds up and swirls around me, creating a barrier of positivity. With this visualization I imagine a protective barrier no amount of negative energy or toxic behavior can penetrate. It helps me feel as if I've given myself a boost of life and protected my good energy.

manifestation visualization

If you desire something specific to come into your life, try this: conjure up the sensation of what achieving it would feel like, visualize yourself in that circumstance, and make yourself as physically and spiritually open as possible for it to happen. You'll start to see that what you spend time manifesting and focusing on actually comes to fruition for you. But remember to focus on the feeling it gives you, not on how you think it will look. Meaning, imagine how you will feel in that moment rather than picturing how it will go from an outsider's perspective, as if you're watching it on TV.

MANTRAS

The word *mantra* comes together from two words: *man*, which means "mind," and *tra*, which means "transport." The idea is to focus on a specific mantra (for example: *I am strong* or *I am organized*) as a way to strengthen your thoughts and fuel your intentions. I like working with affirmations when it comes to practicing mantras. Often I'll leave myself a note with an affirmation on my bathroom mirror or on the dashboard of my car. To me it's about setting your energy forth in the direction of what you want to be achieving. You're assisting your spiritual and emotional growth by constantly reminding yourself of how you intend to feel.

Affirmations are not productive if you're trying to tell yourself something you don't necessarily believe. For example, during a breakup, a nonproductive mantra would be *I am over him*. If you're in a sad place, repeating the words *I am so happy* is not going to suddenly make you a happier person. But change those mantras to *I love myself* or *I value my strength as a woman*, and now we're talking. Mantras are supposed to be about something deeper, beyond the surface of any situation. They're about the root of who you are and where your journey will lead you.

Sometimes I close my eyes for a few minutes and I repeat a mantra in my head while taking deep, purposeful breaths. Instead of sitting in silence or just listening to your breath, it is sometimes more productive to repeat an affirmation.

I suggest working on each mantra for a minimum of one week. You'll know when it's time to switch it up. Keep in mind there is not a timeline or schedule to stick to. It's about growing with yourself and setting your energy forth in the direction of what you want to be achieving.

Don't know where to start? Some of my favorite affirmations or mantras include:

I listen to my heart.

I trust myself.

I am powerful and connected.

Also, one of my favorite mantras that will almost always create a breakthrough is *Ho'oponopono*. It means "I'm sorry. I forgive you. I love you. Thank you."

An ayurvedic mantra I use a lot is *Om namah shivaya*, a very powerful mantra for healing. Everly and I sometimes sing it while in the shower or during bath time. She thinks it makes her magical powers stronger, and of course I agree.

OUTER BEAUTY

My mom always taught me to value my skin and appreciate quality products. She has no issue with investing in hundred-dollar creams and retinol. She has always taken the time to really take care of her skin, and she passed this down to me. When I was a teenager, I started to complain about my skin getting congested after all the heavy dance-competition makeup. That and an overall lackluster complexion that seemed pale and dull, at least to me. Mom took me to the depart-ment store and introduced me to Clinique toner and moisturizer. I watched my skin get brighter and clearer once I gave it a little TLC. She also taught me early on the importance of treating not only my face but also my hands and neck.

I learned later on about the power of oils, especially argan and rose. People are afraid to use oil on their faces because they think it will result in clogged pores, but oils are actually extremely soothing, hydrating, and antiaging. And as a bonus, you walk around smelling like a spa!

I didn't get acne until I was in my twenties. It came completely out of the blue. In an attempt to get rid of the acne scars, I went in for an ablative laser treatment I had gotten a coupon for in a gift bag. This was given way too strongly and I walked out with discolored racing stripes on my face! Suffice it to say I was not happy. One of the many lessons I've learned is to do my research before making a big decision. The laser triggered something, and as a result I have since spent my life battling melasma, dark brown patches that appear on my face. The negative side of dealing with the discoloration is that I'm constantly fighting it. The silver lining is I go in often for facials, try all the new beauty treatments, and have become a bona fide frustrated esthetician. And I have found that researching and learning about this mediscience world is something I love to do.

So what have I learned after a decade of trial and error? Well, all the fancy gadgets and new treatments can work temporarily, but it really is about consistency and staying on top of a skin regimen as much as you can. It's also about giving yourself a break, loving your imperfections, and realizing there are no quick fixes. I am a huge fan of microdermabrasion, a treatment that essentially sands off dead skin cells. I swear by this service. It's so good for your skin to turn over new cells. I also use kojic acid and brightening products like licorice root and Pitera. Some skin products you need to use for a period of time and then take a break and try a new serum. It's all a learning process.

But because I don't want to compromise the services I invest in, I'm very good about washing my face at night. It sounds basic but it's key. Even when I've had too many cocktails or filmed an all-nighter and can barely make it to my bed, I will still wash my face first.

Here's the honest truth and hands down most effective way to achieve clear, glowing skin, but you may not want to hear it: it's all about your diet. When I cut out dairy and gluten, replacing them with green juices and smoothies, the difference in the texture and tonality of my skin is like night and day. What we eat and drink truly shows up on our faces. This simple (yet hard to implement all the time—I understand!) truth continues to astonish me. A green smoothie or celery juice in the morning will do wonders for your skin, energy, and health. For that reason (and for many others, of course), I make an extra effort to eat as healthy as I can, as much as I can, and to serve myself clean greens.

TAKE WITH YOU

Practicing meditation and preparing nutritious
meals brings me so much joy and feeds my desire
for routine. I love to share what I learn and create
with friends and coworkers. Doing beautiful things
for myself is nice, but being able to give that gift to
someone else–well, there's nothing more beautiful
than that!

stop burying the parts of yourself

that you don't understand . . .

the earth will just keep returning them until you plant them into something that

will grow.

— APRIL GREEN

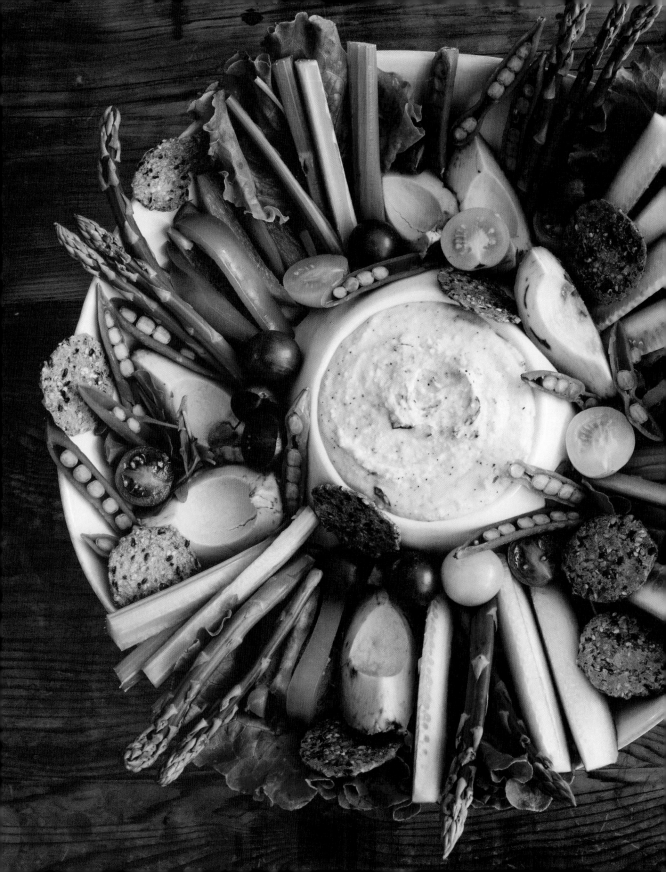

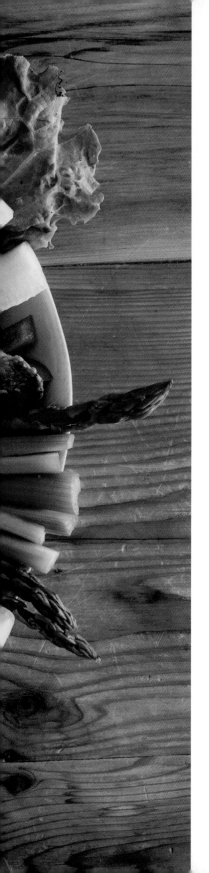

CHAPTER FOUR

plant life

As a kid, I never really liked the taste of meat. I had a pretty good idea of where it came from, and it didn't sit well with me. In fact, as wild as it seems, when faced with a plate of food I'd often ask my mom, "Did this have a mommy and a daddy?" You can imagine the look on her face as she tried to explain that one. In my preteen years, my curiosity switched to devastation when my girlfriend and I happened upon a documentary on a slaughterhouse. The abusive, inhumane acts so-called civilized people were perpetrating upon innocent animals were incomprehensible. I couldn't believe this was happening. All I knew was that I didn't want to be a part of it. Traumatized, I walked into the living room and declared myself a vegetarian.

Luckily my mom didn't fight me on my choice. Instead, she took me to a nutritionist to help me gain an understanding of how to eat a healthy plant-based diet. Despite what the nutritionist taught me about balanced meals, during most of my teen years I consumed like a carbitarian. Is *carbitarian* even a word? Because it should be! I existed mostly on breads, pastas, pizza, and cheese. I didn't realize that by mostly consuming carbs alone I was actually being unhealthy. As I got older, I began to recognize how dairy was bothering my body. I was constantly fighting upper respiratory issues and digestive problems. When I started researching the health effects of dairy, I stumbled across yet more inhumane acts, this time involving dairy cows. It broke my heart to see

videos of baby calves being separated from their mothers immediately after birth, only to be pumped full of hormones and treated like trash. With that, I stopped messing with dairy altogether and decided to try out veganism. For me it just made sense. Ethically it didn't feel good to eat animal products, and physically I wasn't doing so well with it either. As soon as I became vegan, my digestion improved, my skin cleared up like never before, my energy increased, and I felt immensely healthier all around.

I thought I was doing pretty well for myself and couldn't imagine how I could possibly step my nourishment game up even more, but that all changed when I met nutritionist Kimberly Snyder. Kimberly was on the set of *21 Jump Street* working with Jonah Hill, who was on his own health and nutrition journey. When she began to work with Channing as well, Kimberly and I struck up a friendship, and soon after, we started working together, too. Unlike with the nutritionist I saw as a preteen, I chose to heed every bit of advice Kimberly offered, which included eating healthier grains, increasing my intake of protein-packed beans, and making sure my food combinations were on point. One of the best lessons she taught me was about the importance of combining foods to maximize their beneficial properties. Kimberly imparted a very evolved, comprehensive view on how to be a healthy vegan. It completely changed the way I look at the food I choose to put in my body. The best I've ever felt was when I ate Kimberly's way, and to this day I start every day with one of her Glowing Green Smoothies.

It was always my goal as a mother to raise Everly on a healthy diet. I never wanted to push my beliefs on her, but I wanted her to enjoy vegetarian options, be open to trying new things, and always give peas a chance. I began by introducing her to some basic and healthy staples, and when she was eight months old, we discovered she loved steamed zucchini—in fact, she couldn't get enough. Needless to say, I was thrilled. I hope it sticks and that she continues to prefer healthy options. Or at least keep craving

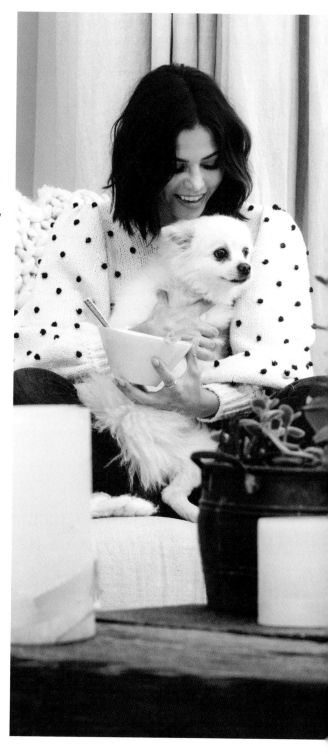

zucchini until she's old enough to order pizza! What has worked for me in raising a strong-willed five-year-old is always having healthy options in the house and leading by example, not through persuasion. But that doesn't mean ice cream, cookies, and birthday party treats are a no-go. If she wants it, she's able to indulge. She's a kid, after all! As she gets older, my influence competes more and more with that of friends. I've learned to become more relaxed when it comes to her habits and to accept the balance that comes with being a modern-day kid.

Living a plant-based life comes with many perks, but one of them came unexpectedly to me. I learned that, much like aromatherapy, consuming certain plants, herbs, and fruits can actually help us heal emotionally from a variety of ills such as heartbreak, anxiety, sadness, and so on. The phrase "emotional eating" gets thrown around a lot. Face-diving into a bag of potato chips post-breakup is not where I'm going with this. Sure, you can dig into a sweet or savory dish in an attempt to fill an emotional void, but before you go down that delicious rabbit hole, consider the simpler (less regrettable) route. For example, did you know tart cherry juice helps with sleeplessness? Or that celery actually eases stress? For a long time, I didn't. But now that I do, I work these and other ingredients into my menu to holistically help with anything emotional I might be working through. Oftentimes we aren't aware of how gentle approaches can actually be wonderfully powerful.

HEART HEALING: HOLY BASIL

It's no secret: I went through a major breakup last year. Getting a divorce was never on my docket of dreams but alas, here I am, learning and growing through one. In the beginning, I turned to the typical remedies. I drank a whole lot of wine with friends. I had many moments of deep, painful, big cries. And both were very necessary in getting me to the next hour, through the day, on to another week. But what was also very necessary was doing the real work. I had to acknowledge my truth: I was truly in a sink-or-swim situation. I knew my choices were to wallow in the past, put on a happy face and hum along, or face the music by dealing directly with my new reality. I chose to address my divorce head-on rather than push my feelings away, which was a challenge for me because I typically live like a hummingbird, buzzing happily above it all. Rather than hitting fast-forward I knew I'd need to take my time through this change, digging deeply, accepting every little thing in slow, intentional steps. My goal was to get through each stage of loss—the sadness, the denial, and the anger—with grace and dignity. I knew that if I raced through to the other side of the tunnel, I'd never truly move past what was written on its walls or learn the lessons my soul so desperately wanted me to learn.

The process wasn't cute, light, or fluffy. It was a dark and difficult time, for sure. What really helped me through the worst days was the thought that maybe I was being broken apart to be put back together, but this time in a better way.

These trials are tough, but they are also part of the life we were given. We should use them to our advantage so that when we do come out of the tunnel, we are better off than when we began the journey. My advice to anyone going through heartbreak is this: acknowledge your emotions and do the work. Meet with a therapist, look into breathwork, meditate, take walks in nature, and have wine with your friends. If you don't transmute your feelings, you transmit them to others—your child, coworkers, total strangers. There's nothing worse than projecting pent-up feelings in places they don't belong. You have to believe when you are in the thick of it that one day the light will come. There is always darkness before the dawn, but the dawn always comes. Every day. This is not dreamy, wishful thinking: it's a fact. In the meantime, focus on doing the work to heal yourself. This means not pushing your feelings away but working through them, accepting and sitting with them even when it hurts so unbelievably badly. By moving through each day, I was able to gracefully make it to the other side. In the end, you will be a stronger, more expanded, even happier version of yourself.

One of the many ways I holistically coped with my heartbreak and stress was with holy basil. Many people take a holy basil supplement, while others drink it as a tea. When we're anxious or depressed, our adrenal glands (located above each kidney) produce additional cortisol, which helps our bodies respond to those pesky fight-or-flight feelings. Being overstressed and having too much cortisol in our systems isn't a good thing. It can cause high blood sugar, suppress the immune system, reduce sex drive, and create an unnecessary craving for carbohydrates, making us feel even crummier all around. Recent studies have shown that holy basil reduces the amount of cortisol our bodies release during these moments of sadness and stress. One of the OGs of herbs, holy basil has been used medicinally for thousands of years. In India, they refer to it as the Queen of Herbs. As with any herbal supplement or remedy, you should talk to your health-care provider before using it. For me, holy basil was wonderful.

In regard to heartbreak and grief, holy basil plus essence of bleeding heart work especially well together. This powerful healing duo will fast-track you to feeling clearer and stronger in no time.

One thing I wasn't about to do during my heartbreak was abandon the things that make me feel good, which includes maintaining a clean, delicious diet. One of my favorite recipes for stress snacking (let's call it what it is!) is based around not holy basil but the sweet leafy basil. The scent of basil is uplifting and relaxing—it always makes me feel good. Whenever I'm cooking with it, I'll rub the leaves between my hands and take in deep inhales of the lovely scent. The following recipe is for an incredible vegan dressing I like to toss into a hearty salad or use as a dip for chopped veggies. Its gut-cooling and anti-inflammatory properties make this dressing a no-brainer. If you find yourself wanting to break out the chips and cheese, try this first. You'll be so glad you did!

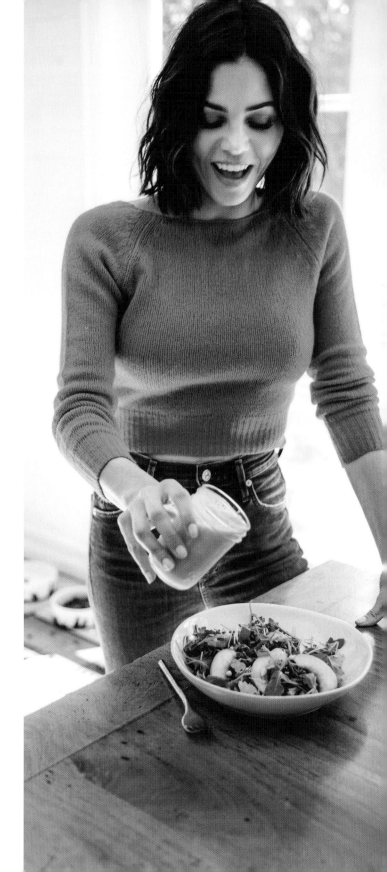

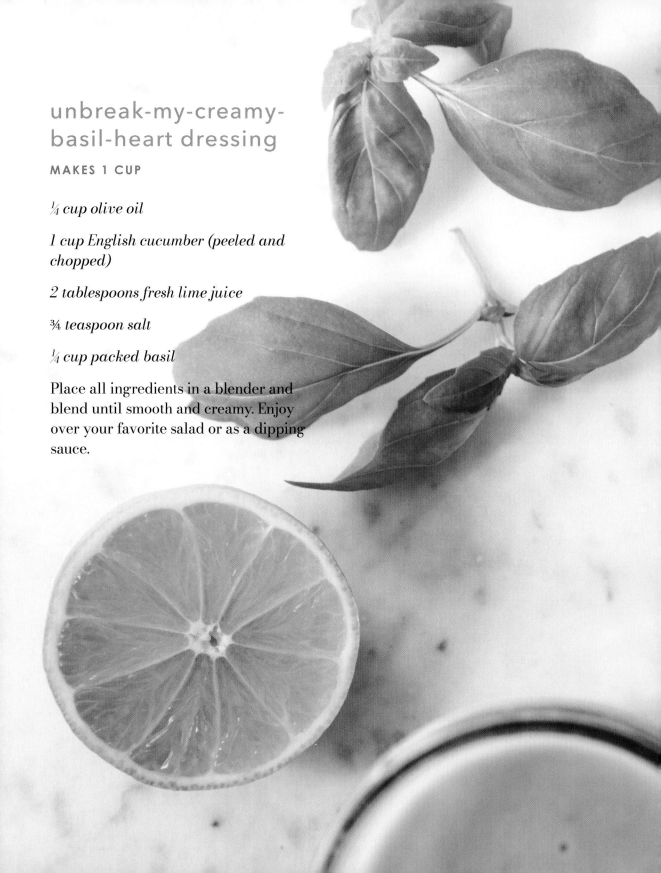

unbreak-my-creamy-basil-heart dressing

MAKES 1 CUP

¼ *cup olive oil*

1 cup English cucumber (peeled and chopped)

2 tablespoons fresh lime juice

¾ *teaspoon salt*

¼ *cup packed basil*

Place all ingredients in a blender and blend until smooth and creamy. Enjoy over your favorite salad or as a dipping sauce.

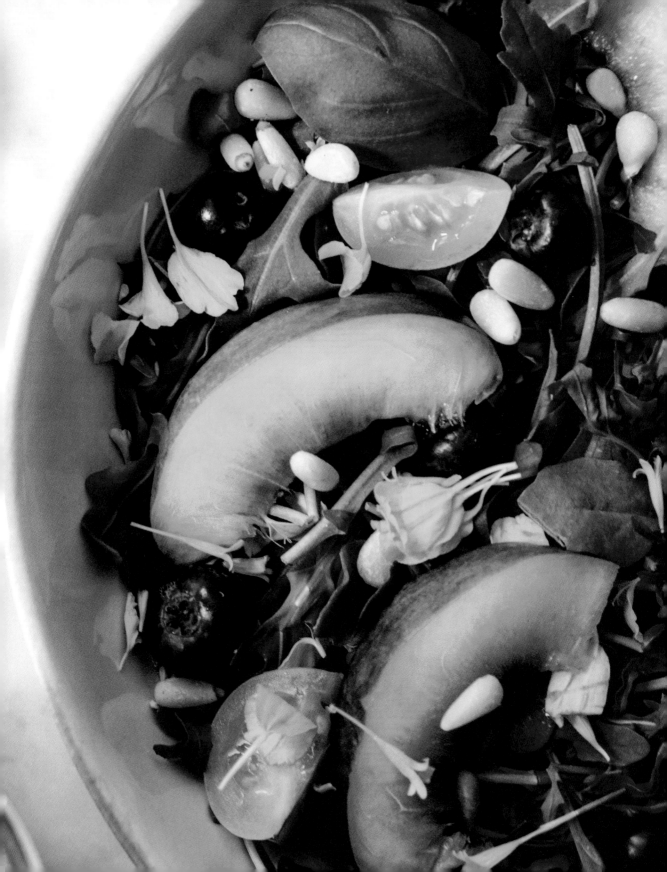

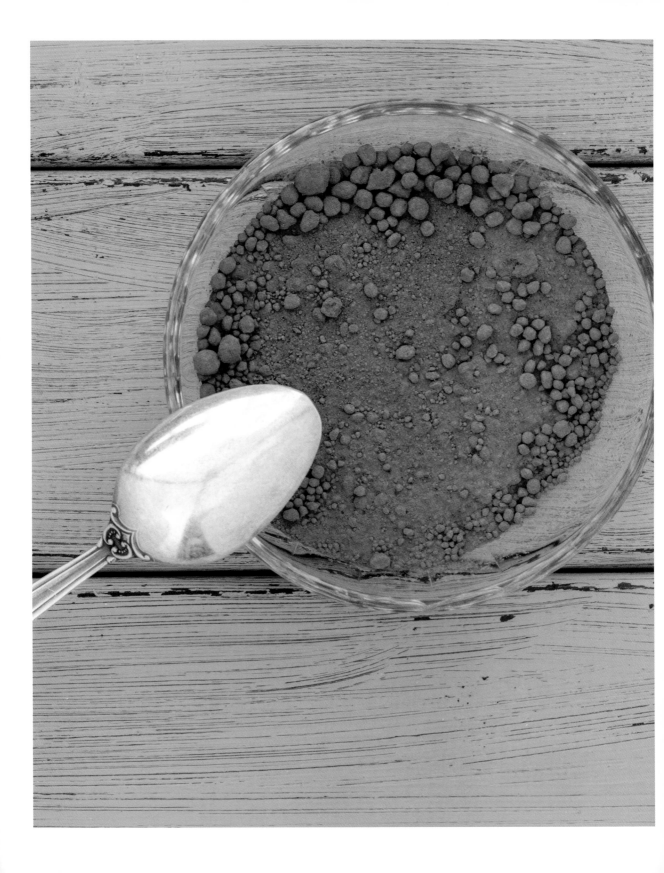

PASSIONATE: RAW CHOCOLATE

I *love* love. I love being in love, witnessing others falling in love—just the mere thought of love makes my heart swoon. From a young age I was always boy crazy. I was that girl in kindergarten chasing the boys down to plant a smooch on their cheeks, whether they liked it or not! I've been lucky in life as far as having great experiences with love. And of course since what goes up sometimes comes down, I've also had quite my share of devastating heartbreaks.

There's nothing like your first true love. Mine came into my life one magical summer when I was seventeen. I'd come to LA on a dance scholarship at the Edge Performing Arts Center. They'd chosen ten people from around the world to come down that summer, and I was ecstatic to be one of them. I was living my best life, learning from the top teachers in Los Angeles. I didn't realize it then but now I know that because of that scholarship, I became the dancer I am today. That trip

was not, however, all about dance. I met Corbin, an actor, and it was instant true summer romance at its finest. It was my first feeling of what can best be described as puppy love. I'm sure my pupils were heart-shaped that entire summer. Corbin was fun and vivacious. He swept me off my feet, taking me on fun, music-filled drives in his open-air Jeep. At seventeen, I thought, *This is it. I found my person, the be-all and end-all of my life!* When I returned home, Corbin and I kept in touch. He sent me flowers and we wrote love letters. But then, one day, I realized I was seventeen and became distracted by very important things like the prom. And in a breath I went from the best feeling in the world to the absolute worst. I thought I could never in a million years love again. Who would want to, if this bottom-of-the-well feeling was all you were left with in the end?

Of course, as much as I doubted and feared that I wouldn't, I did fall in love again, and many relationships later I got married, too. My mom always used to remind me after each breakup that less than a year after Corbin I was happy and feeling love again. That's how it works with love. One of the greatest things about love is how it transforms and evolves. It never looks the way you think it will; then it always comes back around in another form. Love can and will happen again. And I love that!

Since I love love, I also love raw chocolate, because it is high in phenylethylamine, aka *the love chemical*, which has been proven to make us feel blissful and full of passion. When drinking hot cocoa, I always feel like my heart is getting a warm hug from the best lover in the world. The feeling is akin to the warm and fuzzy one you get when you're in someone's arms for the first time. I believe the most important love is self-love, and for this reason whenever I want to give myself a little lovin', this sweet treat is my go-to.

love potion number mine

MAKES 1 SERVING

1 cup organic unsweetened or fresh almond milk

1 tablespoon raw cacao powder

2 tablespoons maple or agave syrup or 1 tablespoon raw sugar or ½ packet powdered stevia for lower carb intake

⅛ teaspoon vanilla or peppermint extract

Heat the almond milk in a saucepan over medium heat. Add the raw cacao powder and sweetener. Whisk to combine; make sure the chocolate is fully incorporated. Adjust sweetness to taste. Right before sipping, add the extract of your choice.

You can also blend the beverage to create a foam!

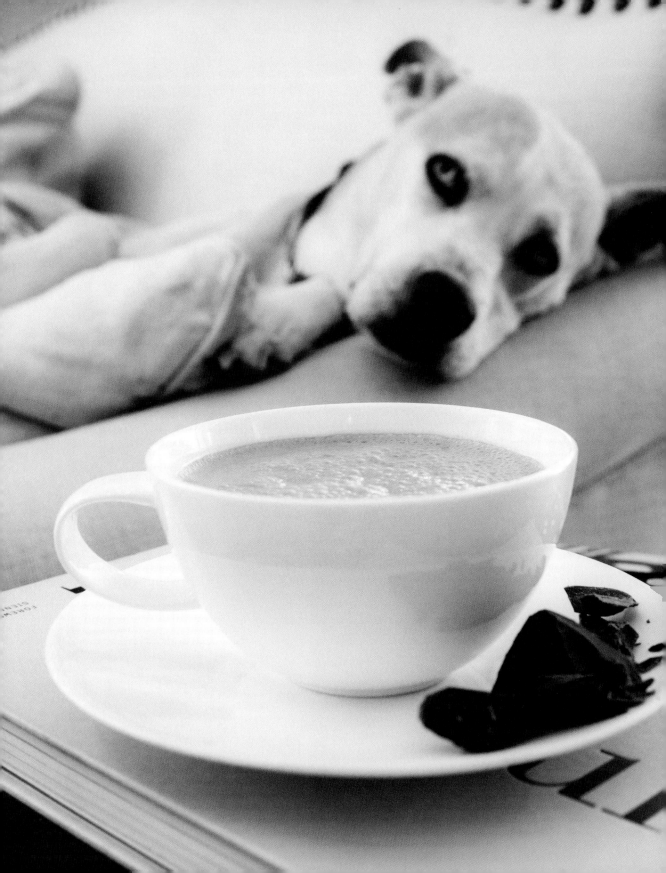

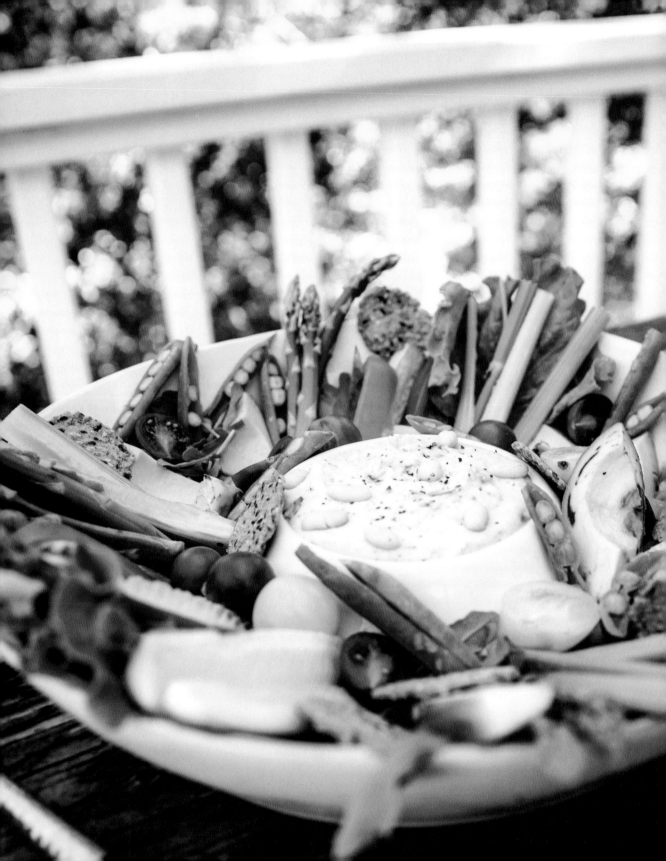

GO-GO ENERGY: BEANS

Our country is obsessed with protein. Everywhere you look, menus and products boast about their foods being packed with the big P. We've been brainwashed to believe we need so much protein, and the truth is, it isn't true. Some nonvegetarians think the more animal protein they have on their plate, the better, and it's simply not the case. It takes your body a long time to digest all that meat. During that time, you feel heavy and weighted down. But when you source your sustainable energy from spinach, quinoa, or beans, you feel a whole lot lighter and more energetic. I turn to beans for a slower, more sustainable burn to keep me moving throughout the day.

One of my favorite midday-crash snacks is a scoop of hummus. Not just any hummus: navy bean–based hummus. Garbanzo beans are good, too; however, they do tend to cause a bit of bloat. This spread is so good you can slather it on pretty much anything! Add it to a sandwich or a wrap, or use it for a veggie dip. Whichever way you work it, it's basically the best hummus you'll ever have.

in the navy bean hummus

MAKES 4 TO 5 SERVINGS

1 cup dried navy beans, sorted, washed, and soaked overnight

3 tablespoons fresh lime juice

½ teaspoon freshly ground black pepper

1 teaspoon Himalayan salt

2 tablespoons extra-virgin cold-pressed olive oil

¼ cup finely chopped fresh parsley or basil

Drain the soaked navy beans and place them in a medium saucepan. Add 2 cups water and cook over high heat for 3 to 5 minutes.

Reduce the heat and simmer, partially covered, until the beans are very tender, about 25 minutes. Remove the pan from the heat and let cool. Do not drain.

Transfer the cooled beans and their liquid to a blender or food processor and add the lime juice, pepper, olive oil, and salt. Puree until smooth and well combined.

Transfer to a medium bowl and fold in the herbs. Cover and refrigerate until ready to serve.

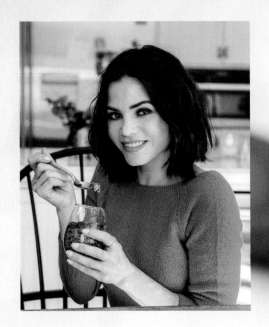

UNFORGETTABLE: BLUEBERRIES

One thing you'll always find in my house is a big ol' basket of blueberries. Evie will eat an entire carton if the opportunity presents itself. Blueberries are a simple and delicious treat all on their own. Every time I eat one I marvel at how incredible nature is to have created this burst of fantastic flavor in such a tiny, beautiful sphere. I am especially happy to eat them by the handful, knowing researchers have found that blueberries may help protect the brain. I might think twice when my daughter requests an additional scoop of ice cream, but I'll never say no to a second helping of blueberries.

This pudding is sure to be a crowd-pleaser at your place. Every ounce of it is beneficial to your brain and body.

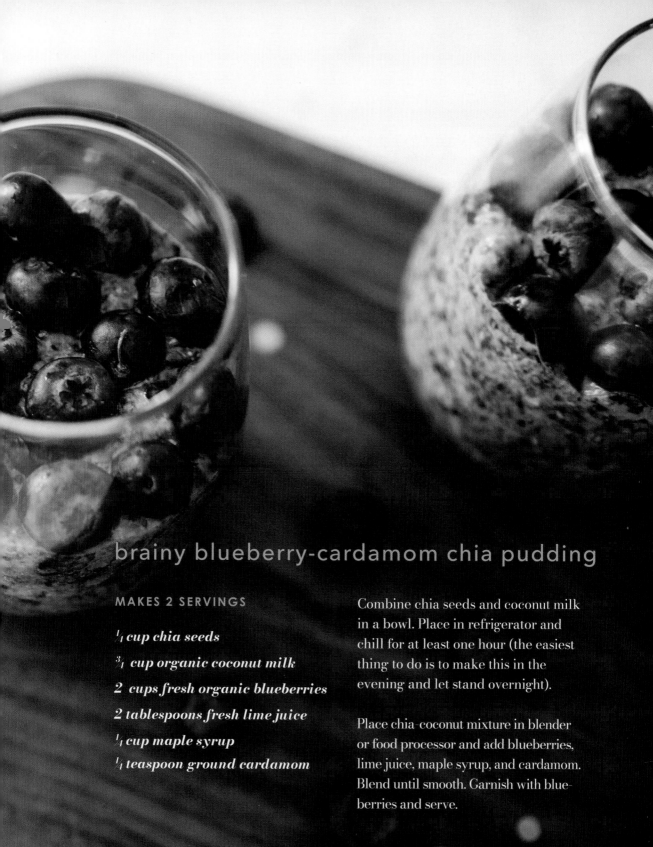

brainy blueberry-cardamom chia pudding

MAKES 2 SERVINGS

$\frac{1}{4}$ *cup chia seeds*

$\frac{3}{4}$ *cup organic coconut milk*

2 cups fresh organic blueberries

2 tablespoons fresh lime juice

$\frac{1}{4}$ *cup maple syrup*

$\frac{1}{4}$ *teaspoon ground cardamom*

Combine chia seeds and coconut milk in a bowl. Place in refrigerator and chill for at least one hour (the easiest thing to do is to make this in the evening and let stand overnight).

Place chia-coconut mixture in blender or food processor and add blueberries, lime juice, maple syrup, and cardamom. Blend until smooth. Garnish with blueberries and serve.

ANXIETY SLAYER: CELERY

Something that might surprise most people is how even today I get extremely nervous right before performing. The combination of excitement and nerves causes my mind and body to react crazily in all sorts of strange ways. I would definitely label myself a perfectionist when it comes to performing, whether I'm dancing, acting, or hosting. Most of the time when we finish wrapping *World of Dance* I get an overwhelming sense of what I call the "perfectionism pitfall." I'll almost always tell myself, *I could have done that better*. But then, nine times out of ten, I'll watch the tape and think, *Wow, that was actually pretty good!*

Fear is just the feeling of having no control, and for someone like me, not having control can be really scary. The only way to get over any kind of fear is by accepting your situation and releasing control. I find that whenever I'm worrying about one thing, I'm actually worrying about something else, without realizing it. There's always a moment when I wake up after the fact and it's as if the clouds have parted. I suddenly get what I was tripping about. Isn't hindsight the best?

When I was a kid, before competitions I would worry so much. I could never sleep the night before because I was so anxious and unnerved. By the time I'd get to the competition and have to rise to the occasion, it would either go as well as could be or I'd fall out of a turn and I would be crushed. I would beat myself up afterward. I would cry and cry, hearing this voice in my mind that said, *I should have done that better*. This is the curse of a lot of dancers and performers. *I should have . . . I could have. . . .* It is very difficult to get past that mind-set. As I got older, I began the practice of visualizing a performance going well as I went to sleep instead of mulling over what could go wrong. I would watch the flawless routines in my mind as if I were in the audience. This practice improved me as a dancer and helped me get over much of my performance anxiety. Your mind is powerful and has such a significant impact on your true experiences.

Training your mind to release fears about the future and be in the present takes practice and persistence. You have to first acknowledge and then address your fear. When your mind starts drifting to that worrisome place, you have to say to it, "I see you making me fearful and I'm not going down this road with you." Put a stop to it when you're in the act of doing it, as it's happening. If you keep looping back around, do something physical, such as a few stretches, a free dance, or going up and down the stairs in your house. Being active always gets me out of anxiety. Movement will get you out of your head every single time.

So what's up with the celery? Whenever we have anxiety, fear, stress, or any other icky feels, they get together to have a pity party right in the pit of your stomach. Our gut holds on to all the toxic emotions we experience on a day-to-day basis. Celery is like a magical pipe cleaner, working its way through your digestive tract and eliminating all that isn't serving you well. For this reason, I drink straight celery juice all the time. And when I'm not drinking it, I'm eating it as a crunchy snack or boiling it into a soothing soup. The following recipe will make you feel good, like really good. Your body is going to love the anti-inflammatory properties, and your soul is going to be light and happy because—yes, soup!

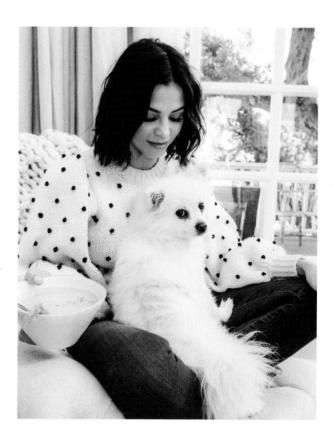

so-calm celery soup

*1 head organic celery, stalks chopped
(3 to 4 cups), leaves reserved*

½ cup organic raw cashews

*2 teaspoons organic ginger root, peeled
and minced*

2 teaspoons organic ground coriander

3 cups filtered water or vegetable stock

1 teaspoon Himalayan salt

¼ teaspoon black pepper

¼ cup fresh Italian parsley or basil

Combine celery, raw cashews, ginger,
coriander, and water or stock in a medium
saucepan. Bring to a boil, then lower the
temperature and simmer, covered, for
15 minutes.

Add in the salt and pepper. Purée in a high-
speed blender with the herbs. (If using a
regular blender, strain afterward.)

Serve soup topped with celery leaves.

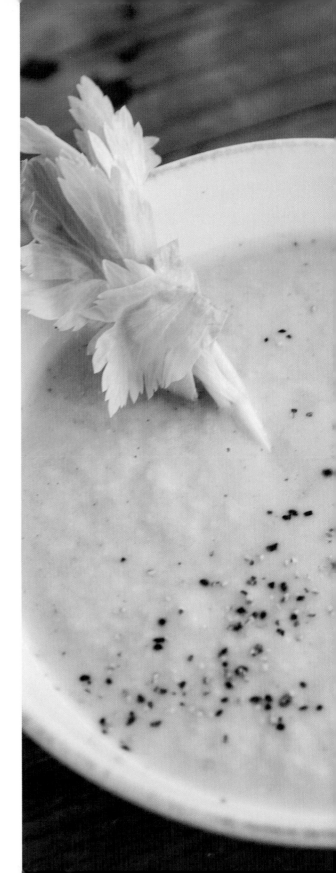

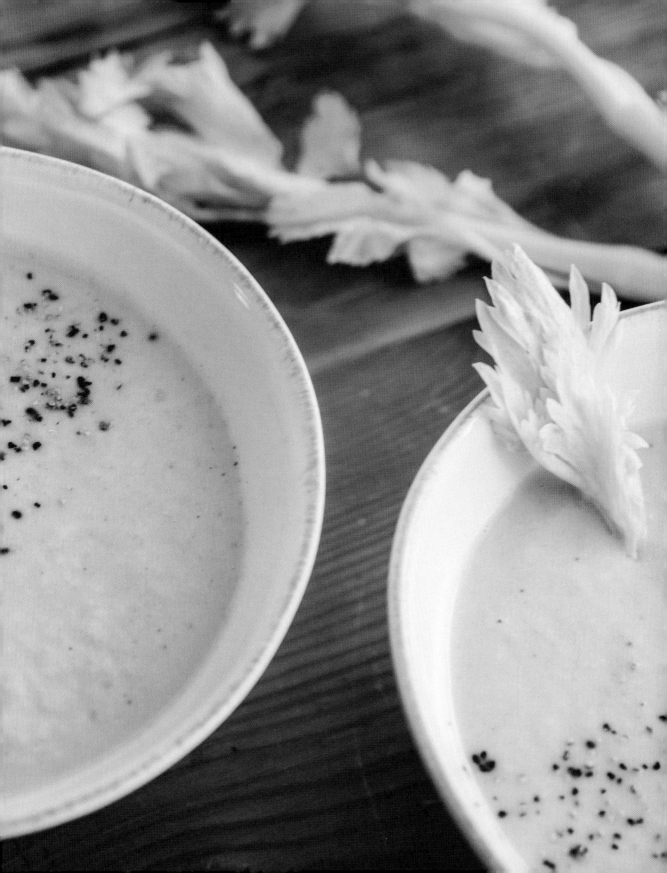

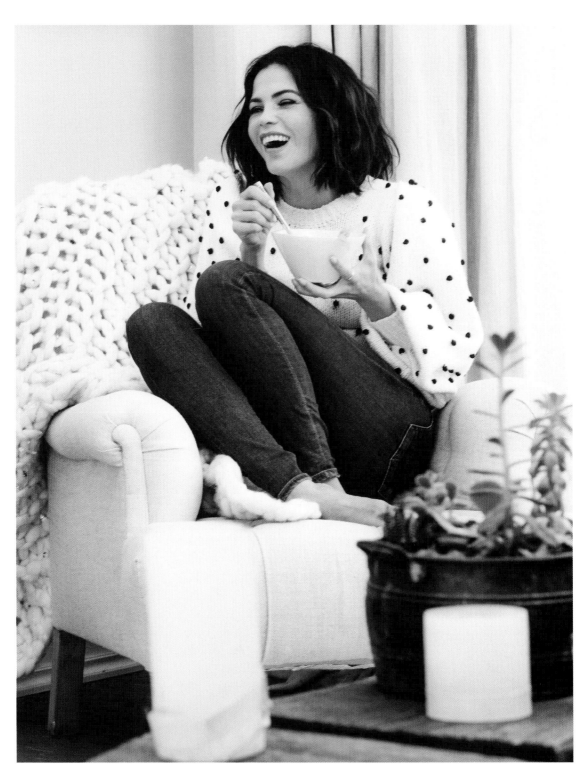

TAKE WITH YOU

Here's the honest truth about my breakup: Yes, I carried a rose quartz in my bra and yes, I took herbal supplements to help me heal, but also my mom flew in to be by my side and I called my friends late at night to sob into their ears. You need to embrace it all and allow everything positive and productive to be part of the process. It is very important to surround yourself with people who lift you up, make you feel loved and appreciated. At any delicate time in your life, it's important to take special care of yourself. Staying healthy has always helped me move forward and stay in a positive light.

I have bloomed and

flowered

a thousand times in

this lifetime;

(even when my roots were damaged)

because I let the dying petals fall.

hope that they will eventually become warm in your

hands.

— APRIL GREEN

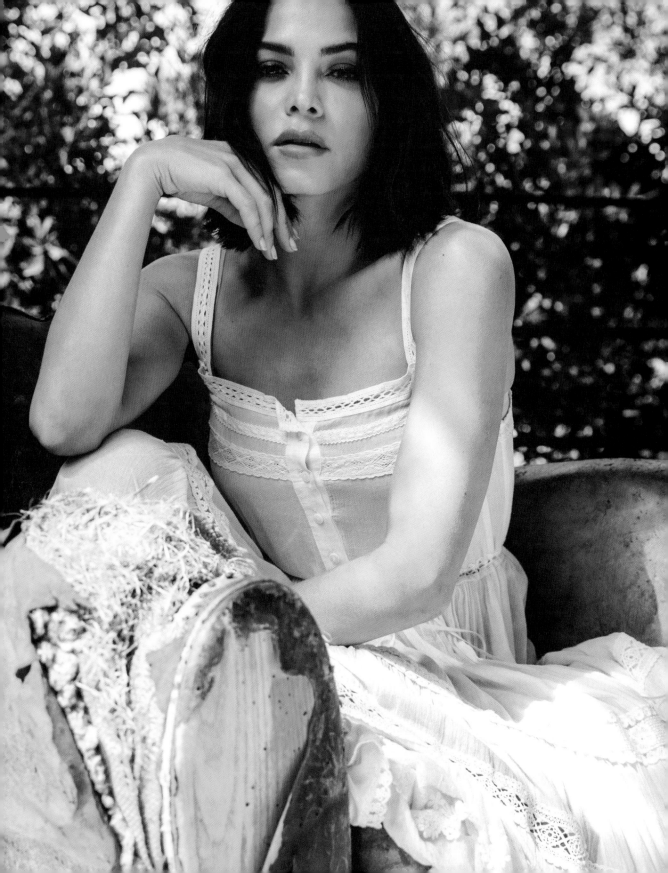

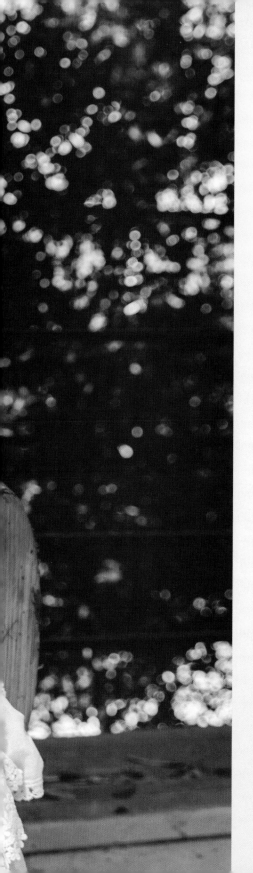

CHAPTER FIVE

very personal style

A google search of my name reveals the endless list of the poor style choices I went through before finding a spot on any best-dressed list. In the beginning of my career I was very "extra." The makeup was slathered on thick and there was a lot of hair happening. I did spend most of my adolescent life in Texas after all. I think going through an "extra" phase is a common thing for young women. Many of us are somewhat suppressed in our youth as far as how flamboyant we are allowed to be, and then once we become adults, with carte blanche to really go for it, we are all in. It was at this time in my life, when I was indulging in all things extra, that I met one of my dearest friends, Emmanuelle. At our first encounter (she likes to remind me of this all the time, by the way), I had on a pink off-the-shoulder ruffle blouse, my eyelashes were curled way past my brows, and I had enough glitter on my eyes to direct air traffic. Worth mentioning: this was my daytime look. I remember thinking I looked super glamorous. On the other side of the spectrum, Em strolled in wearing track pants and a tank top. *Who's this tomboy? I asked myself. What's with this chick?* she later admitted to thinking. Despite our external differences we had an instant connection, and here we are today, still the best of friends.

Since the days of being extra-extra, my style has evolved to a far more toned-down, streamlined, and—I'm proud to say—much chicer look. I'm infinitely more inclined to the California beach vibe, which feels natural and is extremely comfortable. I don't spend nearly as much time as I used to getting gussied up in my day-to-day life. And it's not because I care less about my appearance or that I'm giving up. It's that I'm giving *in*, really. By "giving in," I mean I'm allowing my true self to be represented through my style rather than trying so hard to be someone other than my authentic self. I'd classify my clothing style as being equal parts hippie, classic, and sensual. I feel these are attributes I'd use to describe my personality as well.

When I'm not working, I like my home, my vibe, and my fashion choices to be relaxed. At home, I'm a very earthy mama, so I want clothes that are easy and fuss-free. What can I throw on in the few minutes I have before Evie needs me? A flowing dress, jeans with a classic T-shirt, a long cardigan. Sneakers or sandals. Definitely nothing strappy with a heel. I look for pieces that are actually effortless, not just effortless looking. Some fashions look carefree but are actually quite complicated. I need outfits that I can just throw on and then go. Even better is an outfit I can wear with sneakers during the day, and then put on heels with and go out to dinner without having to change clothes.

My personal at-home style also reflects how I want my life to be lived. I appreciate going with the flow, acting with grace and ease, and seamlessly going from one thing to the next. It's my goal to dress in a way that supports my lifestyle choices. So I can wear a great-fitting pair of jeans with a crisp T-shirt and a long cardigan and sneakers throughout the day, then easily swap the cardigan for a blazer and the sneakers for heels on my way out for the night. To me, this is dressing with grace. There's nothing graceful about throwing things around your closet in search of a look when you're already running late.

This way of dressing works for me because I do tend to be more go-with-the-flow than most people. It's not always easy for people to put up with. I find it challenging to commit to plans and I kind of do everything last minute. It's true! This is largely due to my need to feel out situations and how I am feeling in the moment before making a decision. Am I overextending myself? Do I need some "me" time? But what can I say? It's the way I'm designed.

It's something I am constantly working on. But what helps me stay on time and accountable is having a low-key style. Everything from the clothes I wear, to the makeup I use, to the hairstyle I have, requires very minimal effort, so I can be out the door in no time. Whenever I get my hair cut, I literally tell my hairstylist, "If you cut my hair in a way where I have to style it, there's going to be a problem." I know who I am! I can't commit to blow-dryers, et cetera. I like to air-dry my hair right out of the shower,

> *I appreciate going with the flow, acting with grace and ease, and seamlessly going from one thing to the next. It's my goal to dress in a way that supports my lifestyle choices.*

put a little product in, and then be done. As much as I love makeup for big events, in my day-to-day life I keep it at a close to bare minimum because I simply don't have the time. I have to get it done in five minutes or not at all.

When it comes to dressing for events, it's a completely different story! I'll schedule extra time to get ready and allow my fashions to be a little (okay, a lot) more high-maintenance. For all things glam, I favor designs that have a bit of a "wow" factor, a little something extra going on, whether that be an interesting hemline or an unexpected dazzle. If there's an edgy element of some kind, that's what will grab my attention. I am, after all, the girl who grew up in dance competitions since I was six years old, so it's no surprise I appreciate a dramatic flair.

When it's sexy I'm after, I seek out silhouettes that flatter my body type. I personally like to show skin. My stylist, Brad Goreski, always laughs at me, because without a doubt I always want the length of a dress to be shorter. It makes me feel feminine (and

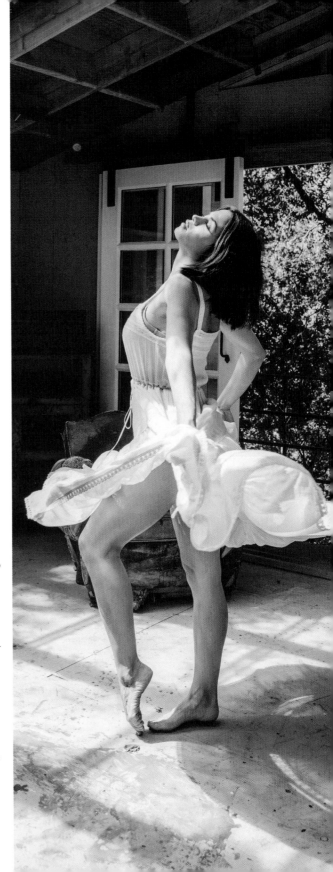

tall!) to show even just one millimeter more of my legs. There are some fashion brands that specialize in boxy, covered-up designs, and those do not make me feel attractive. I see these looks on other women and think they look fabulous, but I know it's not right for me. I feel much more confident in something that show-cases my figure. I think showing skin is completely healthy, normal, and beautiful. We are women after all; we were given these gorgeous bodies and we should feel it's okay to be proud in our own skin. I believe when you identify and highlight whichever body part makes you feel the most comfortable, you'll feel your sexiest.

FAKE IT TILL YOU MAKE IT

There's something to the saying "Fake it till you make it." Sometimes we have to dress and act the part before we actually feel it in our bones. I did that a lot early on in my career, when I had big meetings, which at the time made me feel nervous. I wanted to emit a powerful business-leader vibe even though my inner voice

was whispering self-doubt. To hype myself up I would dress for what I thought the role of a successful businesswoman looked like. Eventually, as I became more confident, my calculated business style translated into my own, and I was able to dress for both parts of who I am—for example, very tailored pieces paired with ultra-feminine blouses. When it's time to bring out my inner boss I will always choose to wear a bold color. Wearing a strong color, whether red, purple, or blue, shows courage and confidence. I'll usually choose a structured silhouette, maybe a high-waist pantsuit, a jumpsuit, or a blazer over a smooth tank top. These styles make me feel in control and ready to take on a room.

I also practice this idea of faking it when it comes to working out and danc-ing. If I'm taking a hip-hop class, I'll dress the part by wearing baggy clothes in lay-ers. Dressing the part is a big part of the equation. The little differences make the biggest impact on your performance. It's the same reason you wear a fitted blazer to an important meeting or a slinky dress on date night. You want to get yourself into a particular frame of mind.

LABELS

There have been times when a stylist (not Brad!) has put me in something and I've thought, *Meh, it's not really me.* Despite my protest, I've been convinced to wear what was chosen anyway because it was a good designer choice. Every time I've gone along with this I've regretted it. It doesn't matter who designed the dress or outfit, it's about the feeling you have about wearing it. The times I've succumbed to the pressure and worn a big designer to a big event despite not loving the way it made me feel, it's always dimmed the light of my experience. I have learned to trust myself and not listen to what others say should be worn, especially since they're not the ones wearing it. I would rather feel my best and make choices that feel right for me than please other people.

Recently I went through my closet and threw away everything that didn't truly need to be there. I got rid of a lot of my dance clothes and loungewear that had been worn to the point of being threadbare. Although those broken-in items were so comfortable, I feel much better about myself in matching sets like my Danskin collection. These items are chicer and cuter than the "past their prime" pieces I cast off. Even if I'm just home alone, I feel better in these clothes. It's not always about looking good in front of other people, you know? Feeling a bit put together and like less of a slob has a lasting effect on me. Although some of the oldies did stay. I had to keep my Hanes men's blue sweatpants, the ones I wore on *Lip Sync Battle* when performing "Pony." They were probably ten dollars, but I've had them forever and I refuse to throw them away. They're the most comfortable sweatpants ever! They make me feel joy. They are keepers.

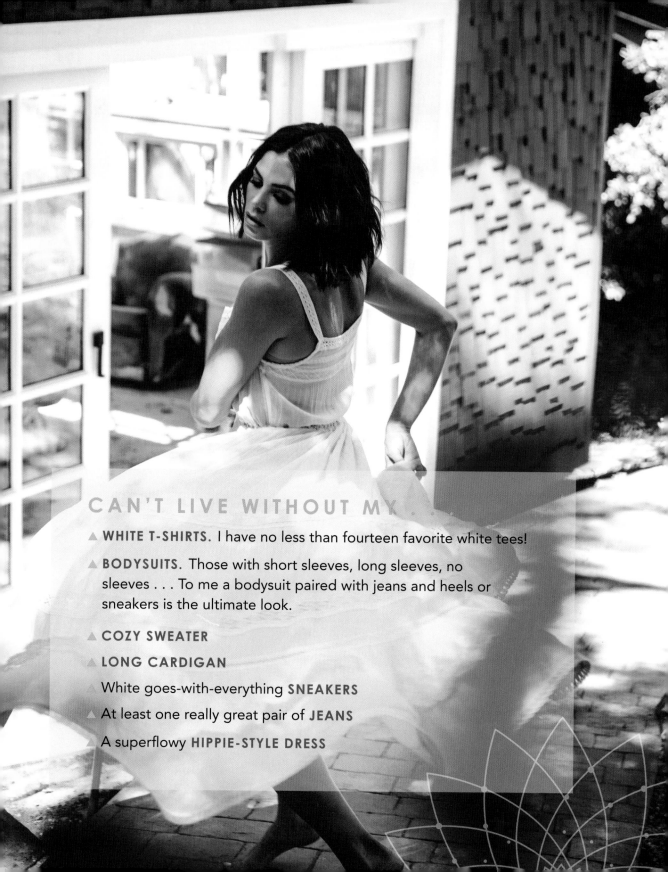

CAN'T LIVE WITHOUT MY . . .

▲ **WHITE T-SHIRTS.** I have no less than fourteen favorite white tees!

▲ **BODYSUITS.** Those with short sleeves, long sleeves, no sleeves . . . To me a bodysuit paired with jeans and heels or sneakers is the ultimate look.

▲ **COZY SWEATER**

▲ **LONG CARDIGAN**

White goes-with-everything **SNEAKERS**

▲ At least one really great pair of **JEANS**

A superflowy **HIPPIE-STYLE DRESS**

PLAYING DRESS-UP WITH BRAD GORESKI

Nobody pulls a look together quite like my stylist, Brad. From him I've learned that finishing touches are just as important as the main piece. Most people figure, "I found the dress. I found the shoes. I'm good." Brad believes the extra details are as important as the dress. Even the smallest accessory can make a huge difference. He has such a big, bright personality, and it encourages me to be unafraid and take risks. He'll always say to me, "Yeah, girl, let's do it!" He's very colorful in life, and that attitude carries over into his fittings and selections. Brad taught me that as with life, fashion should be fun. If you overthink this stuff it takes the fun out of it. He teaches me to enjoy the process, educates me on the "dos" and, most important, keeps me off the "don't" list!

FROM BRAD

Jenna is someone who loves playing dress-up, and I, of course, love that about her. Anywhere she can add some sparkle or go even shorter in length, she's game. I can always count on Jenna's inner dancer to come out to play. She's very willing to try different outfits, and that's what makes her such a great inspiration. She's not locked into one look or trend; she's open to trying new looks and styles. Sometimes these risks execute beautifully and other times not so much, but it's all part of the journey.

One of the reasons Jenna is so comfortable with versatility is because she's very in tune with what works for her body. Whenever I work with a client, we start our fitting by focusing on their best asset. People in general have a tendency to work from what they don't like versus highlighting what they do. Jenna, for example, has great legs and she knows it (who doesn't?), so we often opt for higher slits or a plunging neckline to elongate her body, showing off the parts she feels really good about. By focusing on and working from the positive, my clients always feel sexier and more empowered.

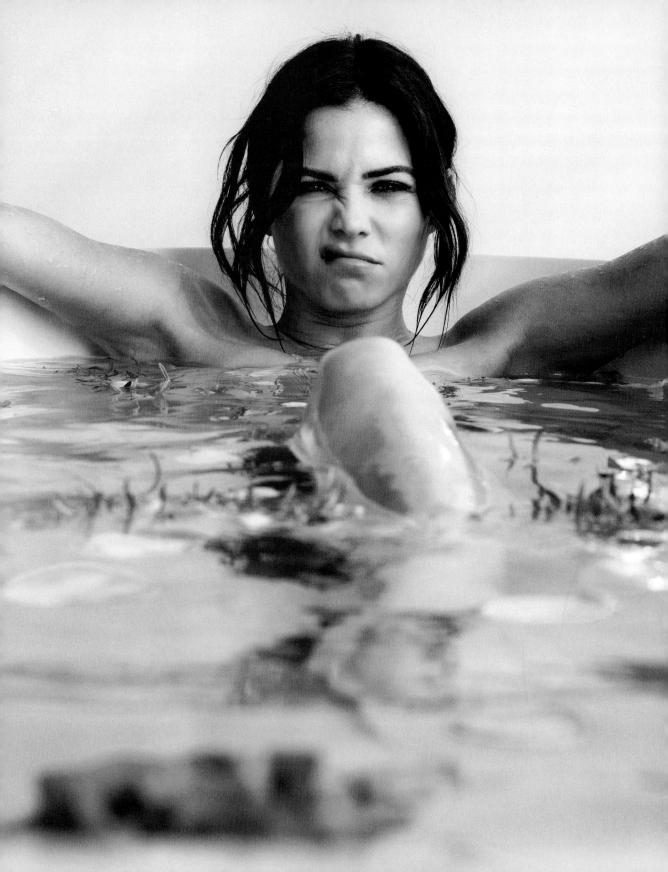

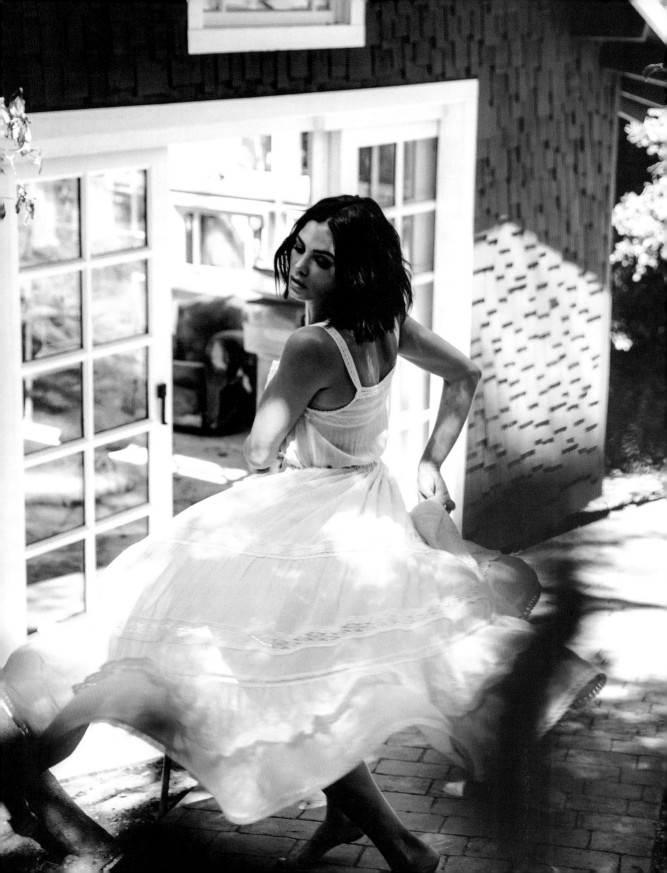

TAKE WITH YOU

In terms of my personal style, Evie gave me the best gift: she taught me to just surrender. When I became pregnant, my priorities became really clear. The stuff that used to stress or bother me when it came to fashion went away. Whereas I used to focus on what I was wearing and how it would be received, I quickly began to think, *Who cares what I look like? I'm carrying a child!* This feeling never really went away. With pregnancy I became freer and chose to love my body so much more. Ever since experiencing motherhood, I don't want to overthink fashion. I am not interested in three-hour fittings; I don't have the time and it isn't my priority anymore. What I was wearing became less important–how I felt and having fun with it all became my main focus. There was a real maturity in surrendering to that.

wild woman—

do not be afraid
to dance alone.

(the earth has been waiting for you)

—APRIL GREEN

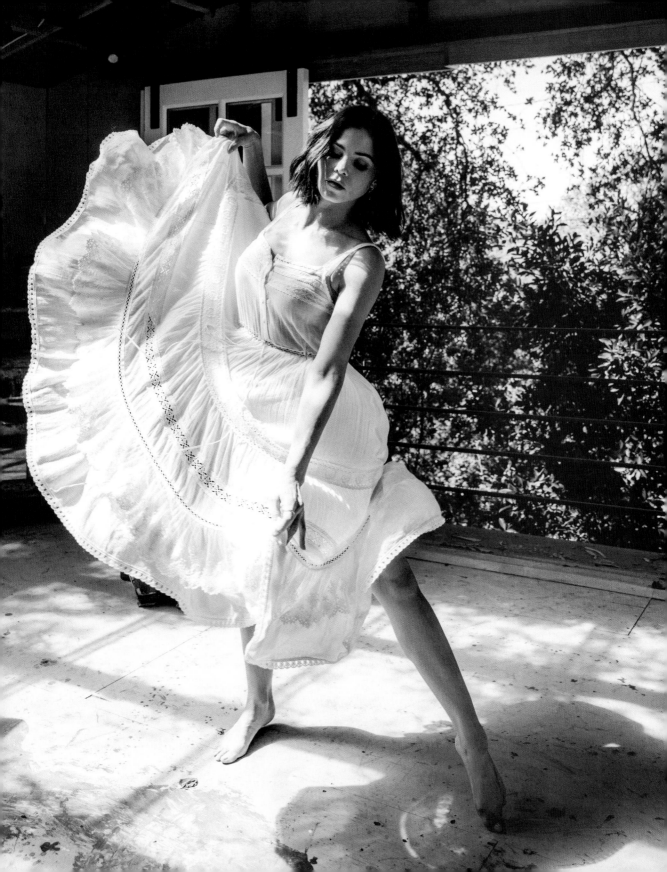

CHAPTER SIX

body work

Our bodies hold all our information—the good, the bad, and the ugly. The body reacts immediately to everything we experience, the physical and the emotional. It's our ticket to absolutely everything in life: health, transportation, nourishment, sex, and so on. Therefore our bodies should be treated with the utmost respect, right? Yet our bodies have been given a back seat in today's world of technology. There is so much around us meant to activate the mind that we've lost

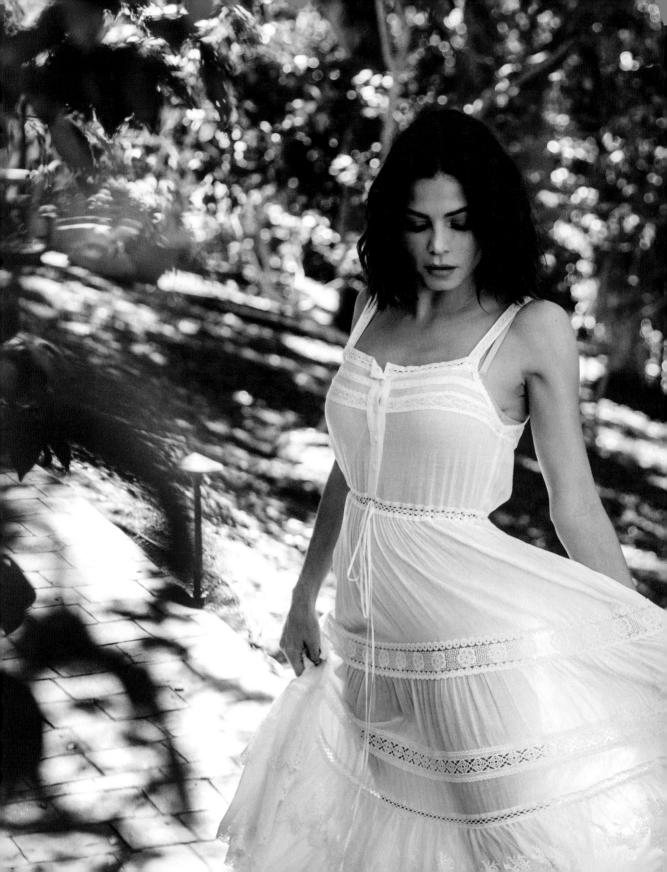

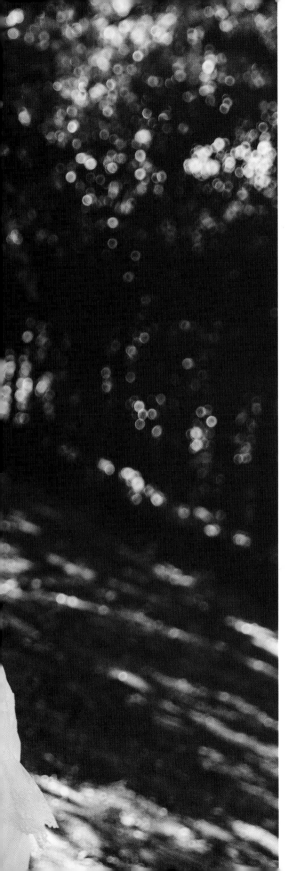

that primitive notion of listening to our bodies. If we sense something is off physically, we turn to WebMD. If we're feeling sluggish, we fall further into the slump by scrolling through our newsfeeds. Those who came way before us made their bodies part of their everyday culture: they'd dance around fires, which they created with their own hands, and move as a way to experience and go through life, creating a connection through their physicality. But today we are in our cars, sitting in our offices, on the phone, plugged into social media, and zoned out. Not enough time is spent connecting to our bodies on a daily basis. We need to connect: we need our minds and bodies to enter into a conversation, allowing both to work together, initiating thought and reflection.

Now in no way am I claiming to be perfectly consistent with my body-mind connection. I, too, am guilty of obsessing over to-do lists, binge-watching my favorite shows, and staying on social media for way too long. When I stay in a stagnant stage for long it shows, not only in my physical body but on a deeper level. My mind is foggier, my emotions more erratic, and my sense of certainty clouded. I've noticed a huge difference in myself from when I was dancing every day since I was five into my late twenties to now, where I don't dance nearly as much. When I started dancing less and as a result moving my body less, I realized how much it was affecting my life in a negative way. Decisions were harder to make, and I found myself way less resilient in the face of daily stressors. I needed to connect to my body on a regular basis, whether that meant doing a three-minute grounding pose or a full-on workout. Getting in touch with my body regularly results in moving things out of my body and mind and into my heart. Put simply, it gets me out of my head. So I have found that if I have something to work through in my mind I'll go on a hike, take a yoga class, or free dance. Clarity and confidence always come to the surface every time, without fail, once I start moving and connecting to my body.

When I was about eight years old, my mom got called in to my school for a private meeting. As it turned out, a teacher was concerned about my health due to the small size of my body. I had always been a very skinny child. I remember wondering if the way my body looked was a bad thing, since adults would sometimes comment on my slight frame as if it were wrong or not good. The teacher questioned my mom as to whether she believed I might be malnourished. This couldn't have been further from the truth. My mom always provided healthy options for me as a kid, and I ate plenty of healthy food. My mom confidently explained to the teacher that I was just built this way. She instilled in me that my body was designed to look the way it did and that it was merely my job to make healthy choices in regard to what I ate. This mind-set created a sense of sturdiness within me, so if someone was trying to make it seem like something was wrong with my body I remained confident, knowing I was making healthy choices and that therefore nothing could be "wrong" or "bad" about the way my body appeared to them.

Things took a bit of a turn by the time I got to college. Cliché, much? Even though

I was constantly working out by dancing nonstop, the most convenient foods at school and on tour consisted of pizza, cookies, chips, and other sinfully delicious snacks. Before long, I'd packed on a good ten to fifteen pounds. I continued to gain weight and soon noticed the costumes we wore on tour weren't fitting me the way they used to. I felt very aware of my stomach, and not in a good way. The insecurity was akin to the way I felt as an eight-year-old, not wanting to be noticed for being too skinny. Only now I didn't want to be noticed for being too heavy. The difference was, this time I had to hold myself accountable for not making healthy choices. A common misconception is that people are only going to feel insecure if they're overweight as opposed to underweight, and that's simply not true.

It seems that more than ever before, there is all this pressure for women and girls to look a certain way. Social media has further fueled this ridiculousness by providing us with a constant stream of imagery that begs us to question our own physicality. Years ago we mostly compared ourselves to what we saw in magazines, where Photoshop was used to digitally nip and tuck the models, but now anyone can retouch their own photos from their phone before uploading them to their social media. Everywhere we look, we are faced with a misrepresentation of reality—and it's messing with our heads!

SOCIAL (MEDIA) DISTORTION

Oddly, body types trend just as fashions do. One day it's all about being curvy and voluptuous; then the next season collarbones are all the rage. Our culture is constantly trying to tell us we are too big here, too small there, too tall, too short, and so on. People might see me naked on a magazine cover or posing on a red carpet and assume I don't know what it's like to feel insecure. This couldn't be further from the truth. Don't let my highlighted Instagram feed fool you! Of course there are things I wish I could tweak and change about my physical self. Everybody has something they feel they could be more

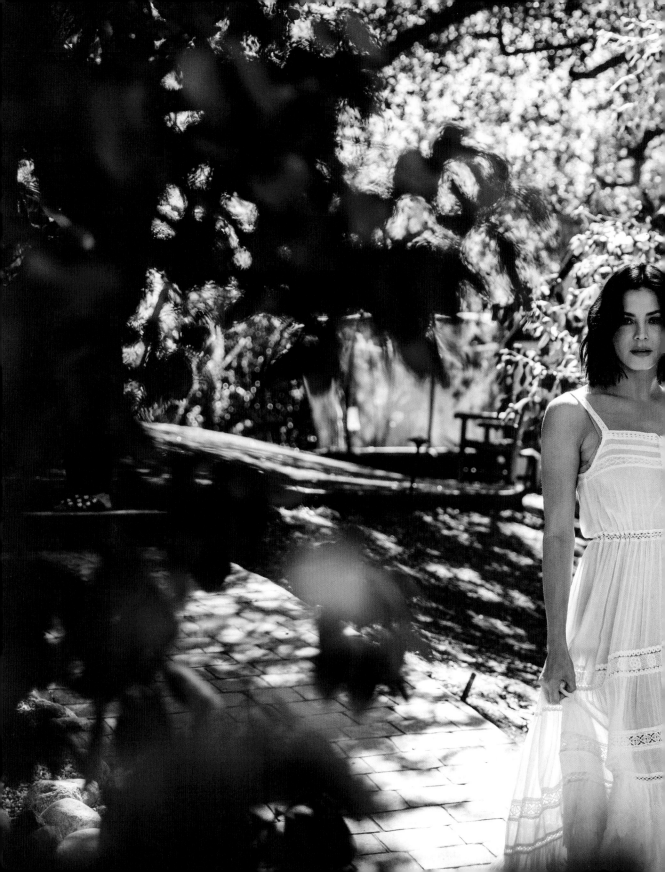

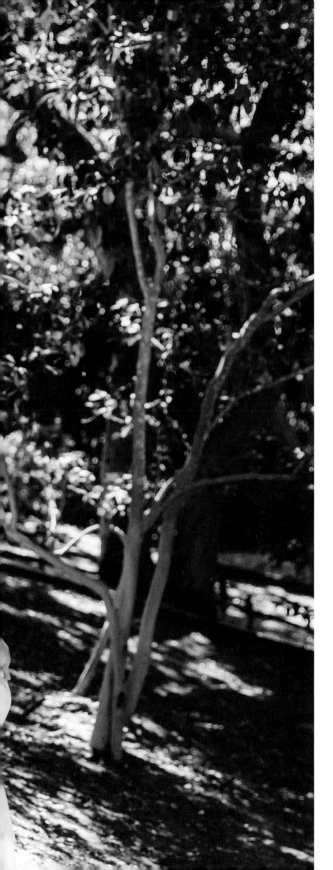

confident about. The best way I have learned to combat this feeling is by focusing on strength, not size. I work hard every day to feel strong from the inside out. Ultimately, what gets us through the icky feeling of not having what we perceive to be the perfect body is deciding we want to be stronger, healthier, and—here's the kicker—less competitive with other women. Once I decided to stop comparing myself in this way, I saw the world around me in a much brighter light. As I learned from my mom early on at eight years old, everyone comes into this world with his or her own unique body. It is the way we were designed. It's okay to want to change what we were given to work with, but it has to come from a place of wanting to strengthen something within rather than saying, "I want to look like her." Body image truly comes from within. Having an inner strength builds trust between your mind and your body, and that trust has a profound effect on everything in your life.

Being a dancer, I was taught from a young age to listen to and trust my body

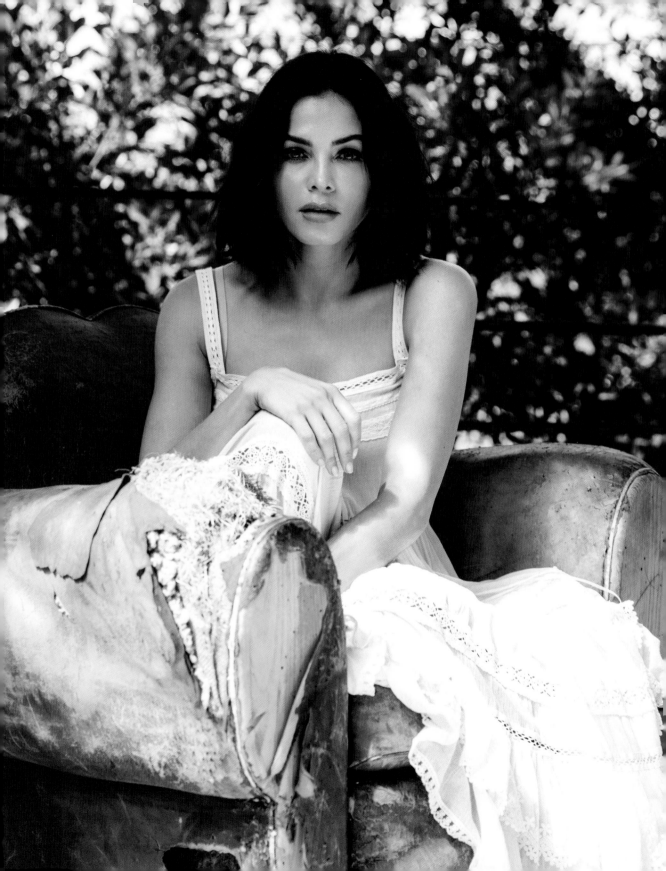

over my mind. While the mind can play games with us, the body doesn't lie. I like to listen to my body when it comes to making major decisions in my life and career as well as minor decisions such as weekend plans or what to have for dinner.

When it comes to making up our minds, we can hem and haw over the *should I or shouldn't I?* for hours or days. Trust me, I am the worst about this. I am naturally indecisive, which drives me and everyone around me insane. We've all sat down at some point to write a list of pros and cons in order to come to a decision. We are analytical beings, so it's only natural that we believe we have to think through our feelings to decide how we actually feel about certain circumstances. What I've learned to do instead, for the most part, is sit quietly with myself and listen, pay attention to how my body reacts. For example, if I've been offered a role in a movie but whenever I think about it I get knots in my stomach or tightness in my chest, I know this opportunity isn't making me feel right. If I get butterflies in my belly and goose bumps on my arms, I know the project excites me in a positive way. If I were to think through a decision and list all the reasons the role in question would or wouldn't work for me (maybe it films across country, taking me away from my daughter for too long, or perhaps its story line isn't something I'd take pride in), I could combat those with rationalizations, convince myself I'm overthinking, or find other ways around my feelings. The simplest yet most precise understanding of my truest mind-set is based on how my body reacts.

the coin toss

What if I told you we've been doing the age-old practice of flipping a coin all wrong? The rules we were raised to follow tell us, *When in doubt over a decision, flip a coin. Whichever side of the coin lands facing up is the way to go.* What if, instead, you sat with the fate of that coin for a few seconds to feel your reaction to the flip? Do your shoulders slump due to disappointment? Does your body get jumpy with excitement? Next time you need to make a decision, flip a coin. If you're feeling disappointed it landed on heads instead of tails, you know you truly wanted tails to begin with. We often learn what we want through this type of contrast.

question pose

This pose can best be described as a way of muscle-testing your body. It's one of my favorite techniques to let my body guide me. Through this pose my body will always give me an accurate reading of my true feelings by answering questions my mind might have a more complicated time dealing with.

Stand straight with your arms to your sides and knees slightly bent. Ask yourself a question. If the answer is yes, you'll fall forward; if it's no, you'll fall backward. Test it out first. I'll ask, "Is my name Jenna?" and find myself leaning forward. From there I'll ask more complex questions regarding anything I'm trying to work through or decide. Be patient with yourself and give yourself time to process

tougher questions. I know it sounds a little crazy, but I promise you this works!

heart check-in

One of the most frequent mindful moments I practice is called a Heart Check-In. It came to me one day when I was out to lunch with a friend. I was really in the thick of it with my separation, and she looked at me and asked, "How are you doing?" I responded honestly, "I'm good. Things are really starting to get better." She followed up, "How does your heart feel?" For some reason, this question really struck me. My good friends were showing up for me at the time. Some would say, "I am sending you love," and things like that, which felt really nice. For some reason, this question, *How is your heart feeling?* was weirdly powerful. It is ingrained in us dancers from early on that the show must always go on. We are trained to work our way through a misstep and make it part of the dance. But in life things catch up to you if you bury your feelings, let them fester, and deny your heart the space to express itself. I put down

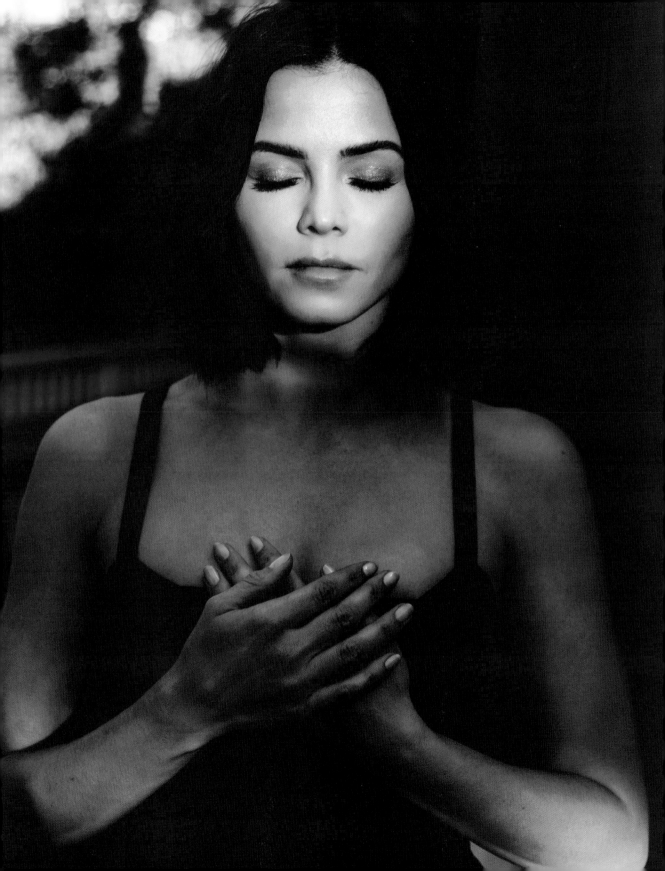

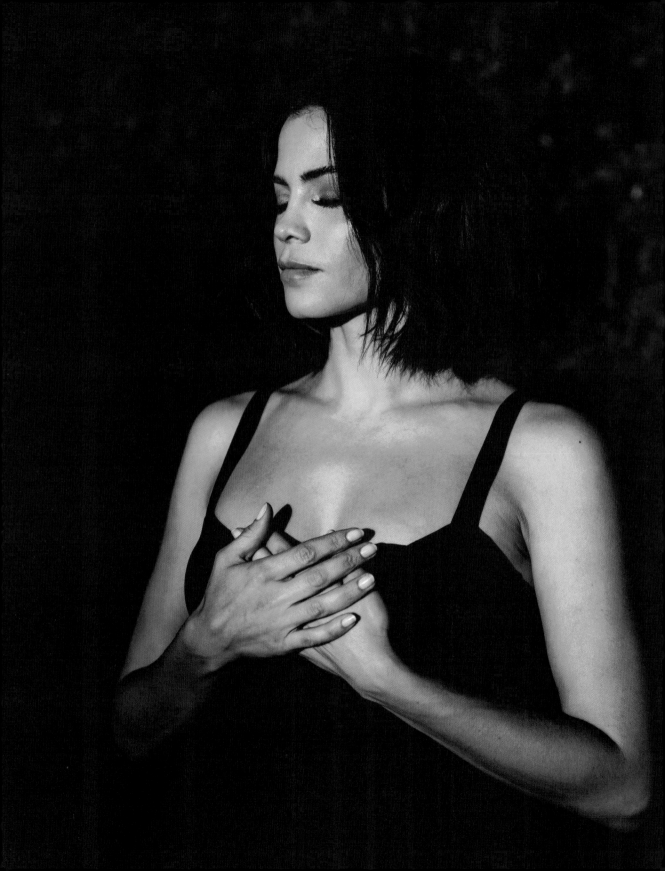

my fork and placed my hands on my heart. I asked my heart, "How are you feeling?" To my surprise, the answer was different from how I felt mentally. In my head, I felt I was so over the situation that was causing me strife, but as soon as I put my hands on my heart, I learned, *Nope, I'm not quite past it yet.* This started a new practice for me.

Since that day, I try as often as I can to stop what I'm doing, even if it means pulling my car over for a few minutes, to check in with my heart. I'll put my hands over my heart and ask, "How are you feeling today?" I'll usually need to dig a little deeper by following up with a "Why?"

Try doing this for yourself at any time. You'll immediately get an answer.

strength in simplicity

I realized the power of simplicity when I was pregnant with Evie. Prior to my pregnancy, I used to think getting into my body required intensity, adrenaline, and sweat. It wasn't until I signed up for prenatal yoga classes twice a week that I realized what body connection truly meant. In this class, we would do slight stretches, gentle poses,

and slow squats, delicately easing ourselves into the physical transformations our bodies were experiencing. Preparing for this monumental moment in my life through movement helped me feel more connected to my baby and all the changes happening around me. I liked to see how small movements affected her. For example, I'd put on a song and sway softly, moving to the music. One day in the doctor's office at an ultrasound appointment, I could really observe through the monitor how my little movements were affecting Evie by the increase and decrease in heartbeats.

In life we often think, *I have a headache, so I probably need two Advil.* But I've found that sometimes simple, mindful moments are often better and can even be more effective. This can mean stretching before a big meeting instead of having that second coffee, or grounding yourself in a yoga pose the morning of a test. Getting into your body yields different results than sitting and meditating because it awakens you physically as well as mentally, then connects mind and

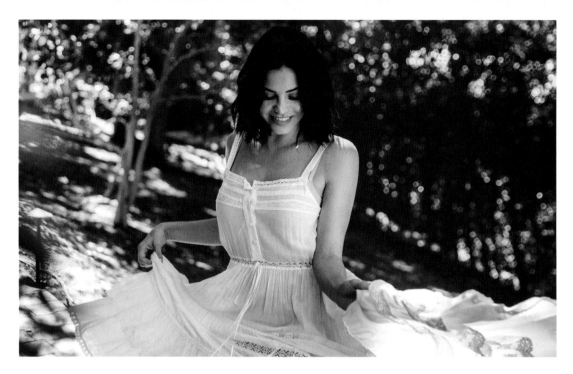

body. I find that doing this helps me make better decisions, quiets my mind, and ultimately makes me feel better than I did before. I refer to my intentional check-ins as "mindful moments," because that's what they are: intentional practices that only really take a few minutes at most. These mindful moments allow me to feel the abstract, not the linear, of everyday life.

free dance

We've all heard the phrase a million times before: *dance like nobody's watching.* The most overused cliché of all time,

am I right? But here's the thing: you absolutely should. Shut the blinds, lock your door, do whatever you need to do to feel comfortable and free, then pick out a ballad that inspires you to move! Free dancing is incredibly powerful. Instantly, tension escapes your body and your mood is completely changed. We can drive ourselves crazy by constantly cycling through thoughts, but it's impossible for those thoughts to keep up when you're moving at a rapid-fire pace. You'll be surprised by the movements your body comes up with when you truly let go.

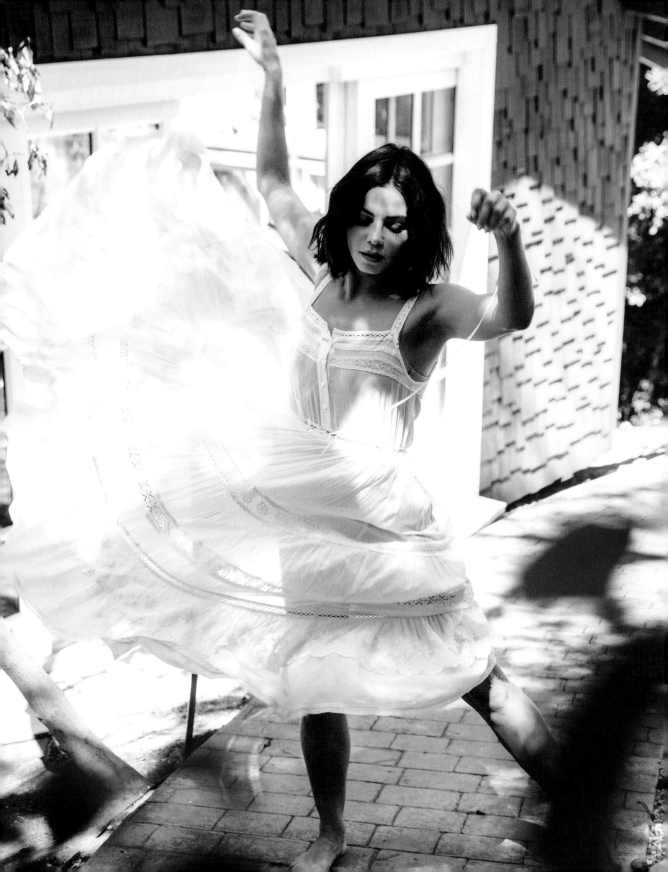

Grounding Pose

I used this quick pose a lot while filming *World of Dance*. I hardly had any alone or quiet time throughout the days we were filming, and with people constantly pulling me in this and that direction, always in my ear (literally!), I would sometimes need a moment to center. Yet often I wouldn't have more than a few moments back-stage to close my eyes and breathe. The good news is that's all you really need, and you can do it both by yourself and even in a crowd. It always works to calm my nerves immediately.

Start by standing with your legs shoulder-width apart.

Take several deep belly breaths, slowing everything down for a bit.

Put your attention on the soles of your feet, bringing the earth energy up through your legs and into your heart.

Stretch your arms up high into the sky and feel the contrast.

Then, place your hands in prayer position by your heart and imagine your feet have roots growing deep into the earth. Now visualize a huge gust of wind all around you. Notice how solid and strong you feel despite the strong winds. That is what it feels like to feel grounded. No matter what comes to distract and un-ground you, you are centered and calm.

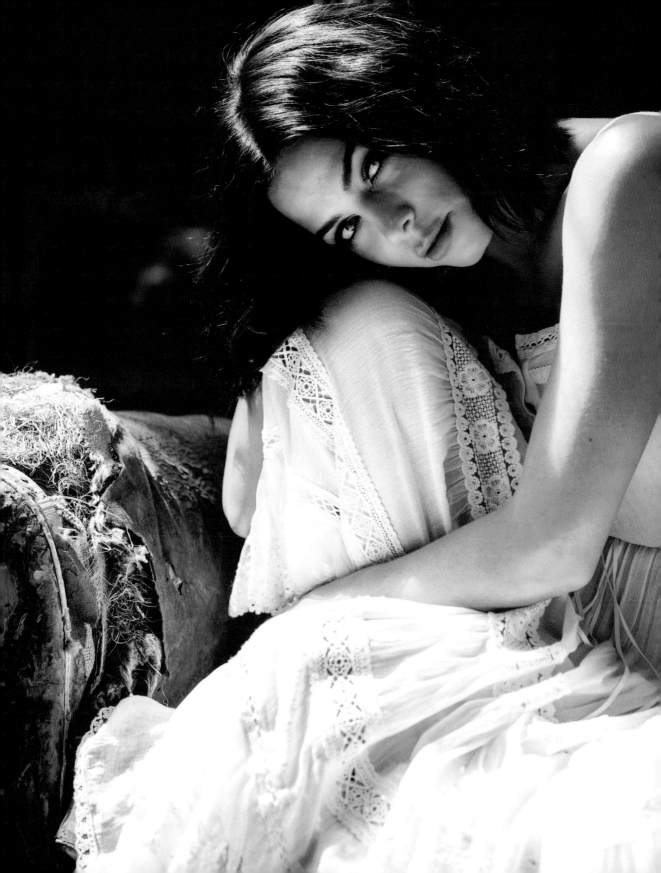

TAKE WITH YOU

By practicing these rituals and poses, you'll find a deep strength and confidence within yourself that will radiate through your physical being. At the end of the day, we can go on the cleanest of cleanses and work out with the most qualified of personal trainers, but true self-esteem begins with how you feel about yourself. And the best way for a woman to look and feel her best is to fill her heart with self-love, honor her boundaries, and speak her truth. I know that when I hold a boundary I wouldn't have ordinarily held, I instantly feel stronger, because I think to myself, *Wow, I just held a boundary and I feel great because I protected myself.* By simply saying, *No, that isn't going to work for me,* I gave myself major strength and confidence that trickled beyond that situation.

Honor yourself by lovingly and gracefully speaking your truth. Make decisions from that honest place, regarding everything from the food you eat to the way you move your body. Choose to surround yourself with light and positivity, from the events you attend, to the people you spend time with, to the books you read, and so on. Continue to check in with yourself, with your mind and your body. It's far better than doing countless reps with a dumbbell any day.

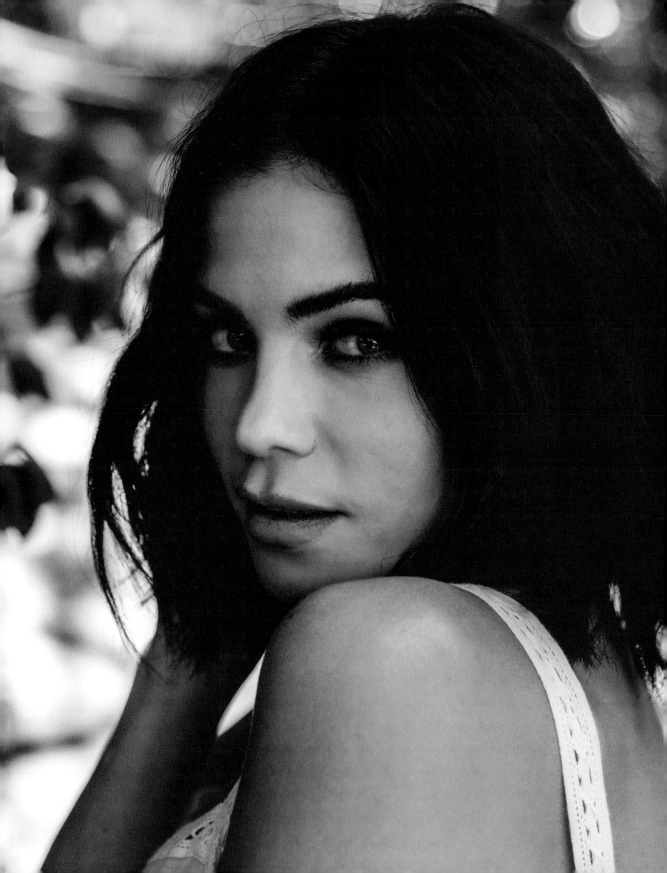

sometimes

it doesn't happen

the way you expect

it to.

(sometimes that's a blessing)

—APRIL GREEN

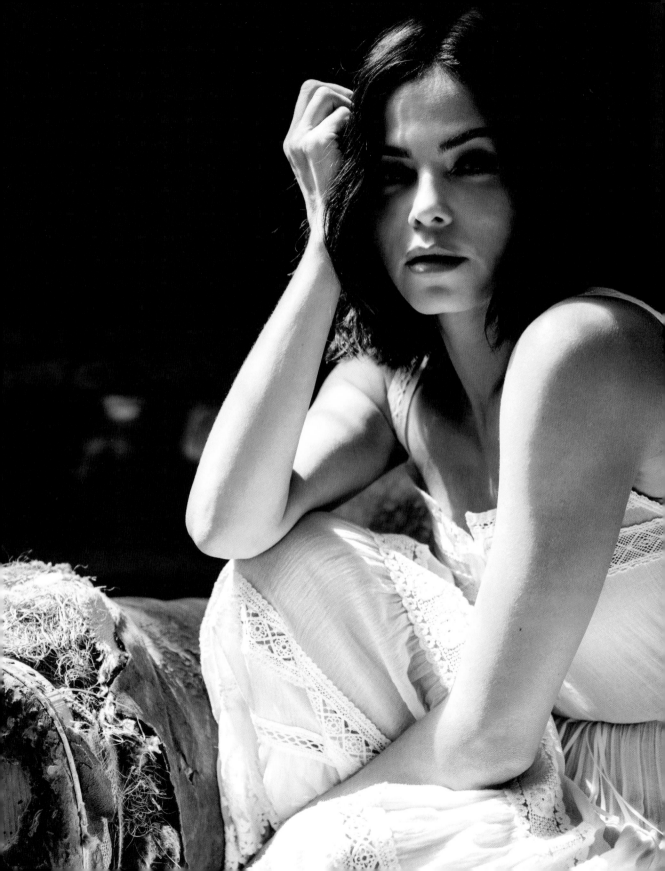

CHAPTER SEVEN

mind your business

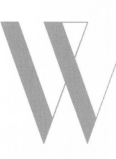hen it comes to working in Hollywood, it truly is feast or famine. You're either working nonstop, or you're struggling to get your foot into any door that will open. For that reason, you have to be flexible, able to adapt to ever-changing environments, plans, and schedules. In this business, everything is constantly switching gears. Where you're shooting, at what time, and when the project will be released could change ten or more times

before anything actually happens. There's no better career to teach someone how to go with the flow than one in the entertainment industry.

When I am working at the mercy of last-minute changes, late nights, and (the worst) jet lag, flipping from Jenna the actress to Jenna the mom can be a real challenge. Continuously swapping hats has forced me to become someone who can roll with the world of events. Right now I am going through this as I film the Fox Television show *The Resident*. Initially the show sent over a preliminary shooting schedule, which I used to plan Evie's appointments, playdates, and classes while I'm away filming. As this job of acting always goes, things shifted at the last minute due to a location change. Before I knew it, the original schedule had been scrapped. I had to move my and Evie's personal schedule around, changing my flight home from Atlanta, where we were filming, and rework everything for my daughter—who always comes first. Years earlier, I might have had a hard time with all this unpredictable change. But after some experience in the industry, I've learned to expect and accept a shuffle in our already crazy schedule.

Beyond having a hectic calendar, I've experienced many ups and downs throughout my career as a working actress. Through them, I've taken with me key lessons I always keep in mind when it comes to my work. By reminding myself of specific experiences and what came of them, I'm able to push through challenges that arise and continue moving forward professionally. I believe the lessons listed in this chapter can be applied to any work setting, whether you're a bartender, a teacher, or a physician . . . or just playing one on TV.

GO FOR IT

In 2002 I danced onstage at the Grammys with Justin Timberlake for *NSYNC's performance. A talent manager noticed me, and she decided I should be an actress. She tracked me down and convinced me I should go for it. I never intended to get into acting. I was very focused on being a professional dancer, and that was where my ambitions were invested. I wasn't sure it was a good idea. What did I know about acting? The answer: nothing. I didn't even know what hitting your mark meant. She finally coaxed me into auditioning for what would be my very first film, *Tamara*, a low-budget horror flick.

HITTING your MARK is a phrase used to direct actors during filming. Often there will be a small piece of tape on the floor to mark where the actor should stand. It ensures the best lighting, focus, and frame for the cameras to capture the scene.

I was truly shocked but excited when I found out I got the job. In an instant, I went from being a background dancer to being the star of a movie.

My character, Tamara, was a shy, mousy girl who got teased at school. She discovered witchcraft (and a pushup bra) and used them both to seek revenge on those who picked on her by savagely killing them. Yup, it was an intense role!

We filmed in Winnipeg, Canada, in the dead of winter, at night. I felt like a vampire, sleeping all day and working through the frigid evenings. My first feeling of *What did I just get myself into?* came when filming a scene where I was standing on top of a roof in a tiny red minidress, absolutely freezing to death. As I was struggling to deliver the ending monologue for the movie without chattering my teeth to pieces before jumping off the roof into a pile of foam, I thought, *This business is nuts!* There is no preparing for this type of work. When all was said and done, I was glad I'd been open to the idea of acting and proud to say I'd given it my all. By doing so, I discovered something I truly love to do. And of course becoming an actress has taken me on a journey far beyond what I'd originally dreamed of, personally and professionally.

DISAPPOINTMENT = PART OF THE PLAN

After filming *Tamara*, I returned to life as usual. Except in addition to dancing full-time, I was also going on acting auditions. I landed a few things here and there, but nothing major came along. I was hopeful I'd get another great role like I had with *Tamara*. Finally, a fantastic opportunity arose and I was thrilled when I landed a key character role, that of Sasha, for *Take the Lead*, a dance movie starring Antonio Banderas. I couldn't believe I'd be acting alongside great actors such as Antonio and Alfre Woodard. I told absolutely everyone about the film and my character, who had a complex story line and was such a departure from who I am in real life. I couldn't wait for everyone I knew to see the scenes I was especially proud of, in addition to the awesome tango I performed at the end of the movie.

We filmed in Toronto for four months, and the whole cast became quite close. We felt like a family. The film's big premiere in New York City was a huge moment for all of us. I had a stylist dress me for the first time, had my hair and makeup done. I felt so glamorous and important walking the red carpet and talking to the press. This was pivotal for my career. I was about to be a legitimate actress in a big studio film! I was so excited to finally see the film, my work, all of it. I sat there in the auditorium with everyone else, watching the movie play on and thinking . . . *Where am I?* The first half of the movie goes by—and I'm not in it. The second half of the movie plays on—and still I'm nowhere to be seen. After all the hard work I'd put into my part, only one or two of my lines made the final cut. I wriggled in my seat the whole time, trying so hard not to lose it. Four months of filming and none of my scenes had made it. How could this happen? Nobody had warned me about this. They didn't have to, really, but it would have been nice. My mind raced through the list of people whom I'd told I was costarring in a big movie with Antonio Banderas. It was basically everyone I knew. I was mortified.

This was the first major disappointment in my career. Once the shock subsided, I came to accept that my being cut from the film was out of my hands and that I'd have to let it go. I couldn't allow myself to take it personally, even though at times my mind went there. What if I wasn't a good enough actress? My mind would drift. I'd drive it back to get perspective and keep my spirits high. Perhaps the movie was twenty-five minutes too long and they had to narrow down the story lines. Maybe they didn't feel my character was as strong as the others. Either way, the big lesson was, even when you think you got this big movie, job, or promotion, you just never know what might happen. You've got to be prepared to roll with the rejection, not only in work, but in life. This just wasn't my moment, and that's okay. If only the future me could have told me in that moment that something much bigger and better suited for me wasn't too far down my path.

NEVER (EVER, EVER) GIVE UP

I'd heard some buzz about *Step Up*, a film that was being cast right after *Take the Lead* came out. The casting director for *Step Up* told my manager they would not be considering anyone who had done another dance movie. My manager persisted,

even though I'd just finished filming *Take the Lead*. The director said no to seeing me over and over again. When we found out my role in *Take the Lead* had been greatly minimized, my manager pushed even harder to get me an audition for *Step Up*, explaining that I wasn't a main character in the "other dance movie." Eventually, the casting director caved and agreed to see me. And here comes a big soul life lesson: you have to trust. In hindsight, I now know I was featured in *Take the Lead* the way I was supposed to be, and that if my role had been shown in its entirety, *Step Up* wouldn't have happened for me.

When I got to my audition, I didn't even get to see the casting director: they booked me with the casting assistant. After I gave it my all, the assistant left to get the actual casting director and say, "I think you should see this girl." Once I was given the green light, they invited me back the next day for an actual audition, a read with Channing. For TV and film, actors do something called a "chemistry read" to see if two people have a believable connection. I didn't know who Channing Tatum was (in fact, my manager had been calling him Tatum Channing the entire time!), but I knew he was already booked to star in the movie. I came back the next day and flung open a door—the wrong door, by accident. Everyone stopped to look at me. It was the chemistry read for Channing and the other actress they were auditioning. They were leaning in, about to do the kissing scene. "Oh my gosh. I'm so sorry!" I said before bolting. I thought, *Okay, well now I'm definitely not getting this movie, because I just pissed off all the producers. Nice job, Jenna. Dug a real deep hole for yourself this time.*

When it was my time to read with Channing, right away he began saying his lines, which were different words than what I had on my page. I was super confused. It turned out my manager had not received the correct scene we'd be testing on. The producers gave me ten (just ten!) minutes to familiarize myself with the new scene. We carried on with the audition. The whole time I was thinking, *There's just*

no way I'll move on to the next step of the audition process. They must think I'm a moron. I spent two hours picking out this outfit for nothing. Everyone was so nice, but I thought it was because they felt bad for me, the green newbie with the worst luck ever.

I was astounded to discover they wanted me back to do the dance part of the audition. Regardless of my self-doubt, I gave it my all. Producers reported back to my manager that they thought I dressed and danced too sexily. They wanted a more girl-next-door look. "Less stripper" someone had said. In my head I was thinking, *Wow, the producers really don't like me. Why are they wasting their time and mine?* The casting director, on the other hand, had my back. She believed in me so much so that she took me to the hair salon, instructing them to cut my bangs and color my hair black. This, she decided, was more girl-next-door. She sent pictures of my makeover and, wouldn't you know it, they came back to say it was too dark, too severe. I went back to the salon chair and waited as they added blond highlights to soften the severity of my dark locks. A week went by and I heard my dancer friends talking about their auditions for the same role in the same movie. I was deflated. Here I was, changing my hair over and over again; meanwhile, they were auditioning what seemed like all of Los Angeles for this role. *What am I even doing?*

Six weeks later I was out to dinner with my roommate. I remember noticing that the television at the restaurant was playing a dance movie marathon, which I should have recognized as a sign. (As I mentioned before, I receive a lot of little winks from the universe like this. We all do!) It was right then that I got the call that I'd landed the part of Nora in *Step Up*! Everything I had come across during the process had been blocking me from getting the part, yet I kept pushing forward and surrendering. This was a huge lesson for me to never give up and to trust. All in all, it always works out the way it is supposed to. Losing my part in *Take the Lead*

allowed me to participate in *Step Up*, the movie people discovered me in. My incredible life path was paved from this movie. So in hindsight, I am extremely grateful for my previous part getting left on the cutting room floor.

LEAVE YOUR DRAMA AT THE DOOR

I've never talked about this before, but here goes. The truth is, there was so much craziness going on in my personal life when I started filming the second season of *World of Dance*. Channing and I had separated the night before my first day of filming, but nobody besides my best friend, Emmanuelle, and my mother knew. I kept it a secret from everyone at work because I needed to focus on my work when at work. I couldn't let everything fall apart. Keeping my personal life private caused me to focus and be present. I could breathe deeper and trust myself more when I was working, because the set was a safe, solid space. Meanwhile, outside of work, my whole life was changing: the stable ground I was standing on had imploded overnight.

Secrets can be so hard to keep. I didn't realize how much everyone wanted to hear about my relationship until I didn't want to talk about it. People in the *WoD* audience would ask, "Where's Channing today?" or, "When are you two going to dance together again?" I had to play these questions off while grappling with the truth of what was happening. The public saw Channing and me in this idealized, romanticized light. This made things difficult for me, because I like being as honest and real as I can. And while filming season two, I wasn't able to be honest. I'd always had the awareness of our public image and felt uneasy being viewed as "perfect." Let me tell you firsthand, when it comes to the lives of celebrities, a picture never tells the whole story. Everyone struggles. Every couple has their issues, celebrity or not.

Anyway, back at work, I knew I couldn't fall apart. At home I was doing the work, going inward to help myself get through it, but when I came to my job, I left it at the door. First, I had a responsibility to the show. I couldn't come to work, take on that stage, and meanwhile be working through my personal drama. The producers and the dancers needed my full attention. There was a great deal of trust, time, and money invested in me. I wouldn't let anyone down. As with anything else, compartmentalizing my personal and business affairs took practice.

Working the compartmentalization muscle during the most difficult time taught me the answer to working through an intense phase of life. Some people think going away or hiding out is the way to go through it—and there's value in that space, but there's also something significant about putting your all into a completely different space. On some level, I think my greater self knew being creative and holding up a show would be a way through the pain I was experiencing at home. Walking into my dressing room, having the happy energy of my coworkers, hair, makeup, and the style team to hype me up, got me through what would otherwise have been a much lower point in my life.

OWN YOUR POWER

It might surprise you to know that despite my being a performer, one of my weaknesses is my tendency to be an active listener more so than taking control or command. For example, I'll often say "I'm sorry" for something I'm not sorry for, and I find it's easier to say, "What do you think?" as opposed to "This is what I think." Being a part of *World of Dance* taught me how to stand in my own strength, and for that I will be forever grateful.

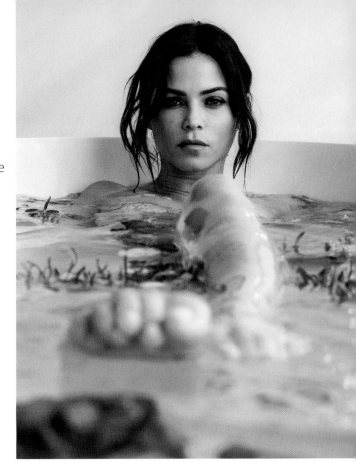

One of my greatest challenges has always been that of actively owning my power. Truth is, I'm almost more comfortable giving it away. Working with Jennifer Lopez, who epitomizes owning one's power, I quickly learned how it's done. Jennifer knows what she wants and she's unapologetic about it, but in a very diplomatic way. It was inspiring to watch Jennifer own what she wanted in her business. I wanted a little more of that.

I challenged myself when it came to my role on *WoD*. As a host, I had to lead crowds and stand strong with confidence, without letting on that I was harboring the intense secret of my separation. It was the hardest time in my life but also the biggest blessing. Every single day I had no choice but to believe in myself. Doing so forced me through a tough time and pushed me past my issues with taking an assertive stance.

ALWAYS HAVE A RIDER (IN MIND)

It's common knowledge in the enter-tainment industry that actors, musicians, models, and so on are able to make certain demands when it comes to their private space. You hear stories of talent demanding for their dressing room only white flowers—or, more specifically, gardenias—or bowls of candies separated by color, or a plate of a rare fruit. This list of requests is called a rider. For years I never wanted to give production a rider because I didn't want anyone to think I was being difficult. When I started working on *World of Dance,* production kept pushing for me to present mine. In fact, they demanded one from me. It caused me to think about what makes me feel comfortable, at peace, and most creative. What would it take to create the most positive space for me to work in? It turned out this list wasn't much of a departure from what I have at home.

It included:

- *Framed photos of my loved ones*

- *Candles*

- *An oil diffuser with energizing oils like citrus and peppermint*

- *Healthy snacks: organic fresh fruits and veggies*

Having these things on hand truly did help me perform better at work. It gave me a sanctuary to feel centered and grounded amid the chaos of the show. I was able to focus on my job in a space I felt very comfortable in. Having healthy snacks around kept me on track in that way. I never felt famished, or had to think about where to get a quick bite when I should be memorizing lines. From this experience, I figure everyone, not only those in entertainment, should have a rider. Why not create an environment that encourages you to be the best you? Even if this only means putting a framed photo of your dog on your desktop, it will help you feel calm and connected to home.

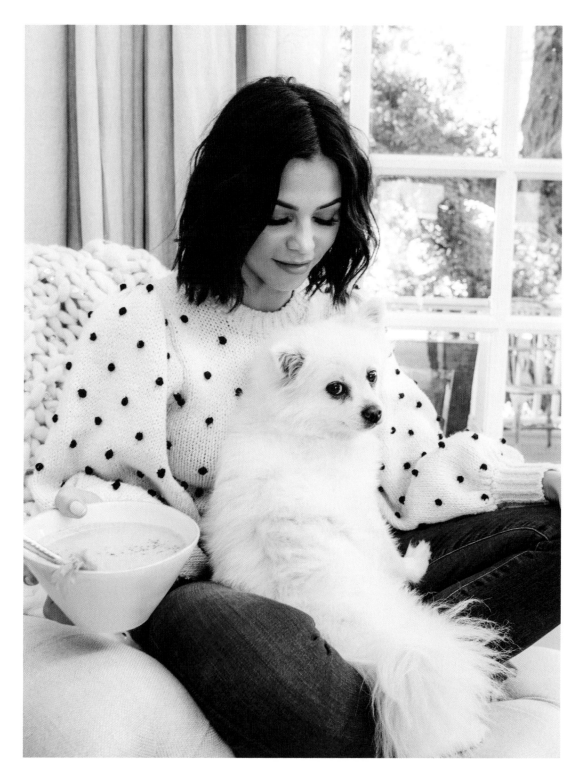

TAKE WITH YOU

Looking back on my career up until this point is pretty surreal. I can still feel a pang of embarrassment or excitement when I let my mind wander back to certain times. If I could cherry-pick only a few pieces of professional advice, it would be these: Go for it! You never know what the next opportunity will bring you, so be open to all possibilities. To do this, surrender your ideas of how it all should look and follow what lights you up. And always, always be a pleasure to work with.

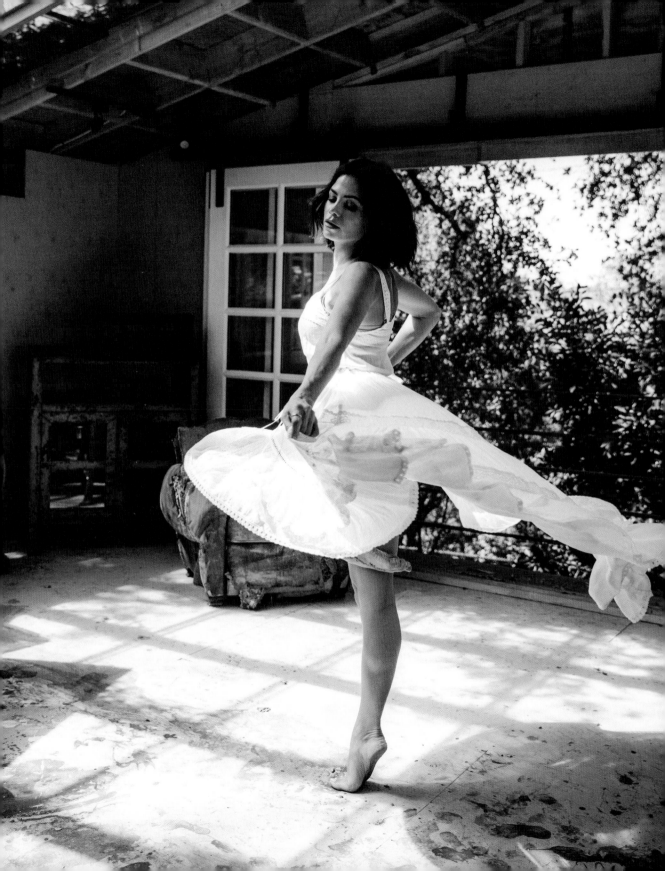

I won't tell

my daughter that

she can be anything

she wants.

I will tell her

to be herself;

and then anything

she wants will float

beautifully

towards her.

— APRIL GREEN

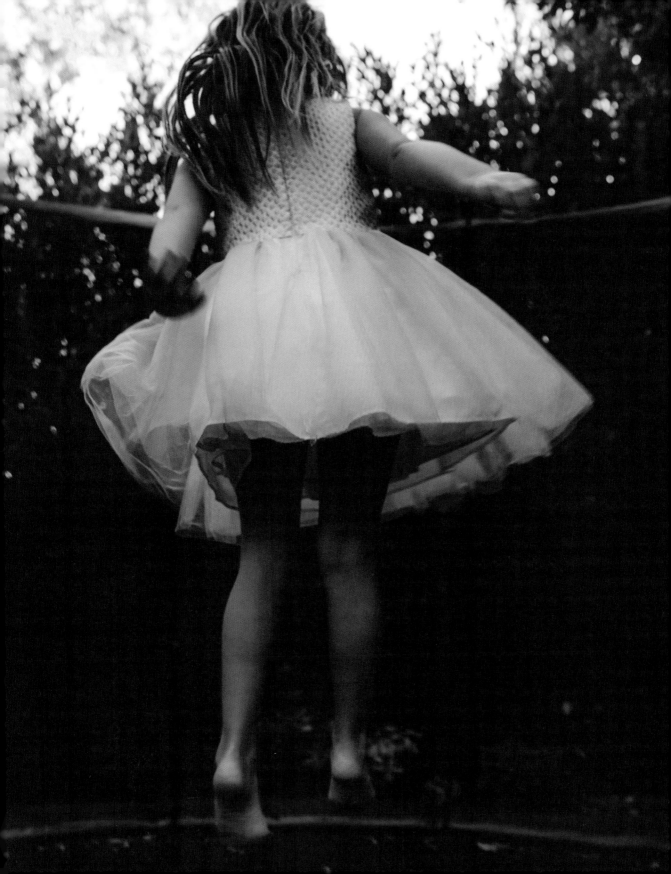

CHAPTER EIGHT

little goddesses

had always wanted to have my own family. Before it happened, it always felt like it was already a part of my story. I famously used to say I wanted to have "a house full of kids running around a Christmas tree." I had visions of a beautiful chaos: kids, friends, music, family members, lots of laughter—the whole thing. Sometimes I think growing up as an only child and moving constantly created this desire in me for the opposite. I yearned to feel rooted along with having a large family. Well, my story is still evolving, but I've so far ended up somewhere in the middle of that vision. Still, the feeling is the same. Becoming a mother is the best, most fulfilling, most beautiful thing that has ever happened to me. It opened my heart in ways I truly wasn't even prepared for. My priorities changed immediately. I became focused and charged with purpose. It took me out of my ego in the best way possible. Simply put, this little being and I have an agreement and a purpose together. I felt it clearly and strongly and embraced it fully. That doesn't mean it has always been easy (the sleepless nights, the colic, the strong will, let me tell you . . . !), but it is and will always be the most important thing in my life.

Before Everly came into the world, I decided I was going to be the kind of mother who lets her daughter be herself. I wasn't going to try and morph her into another version of myself or guide her toward who I thought she should be. As she developed into her own person, I really watched and paid attention to what she connected to. Before I could teach Evie anything, I needed to learn about her. What was she motivated by? What made her excited? Angry? Anxious? From a very early age, my daughter was a strong-willed free spirit with a secure sense of who she was and what she wanted. While I absolutely love that about her, I can't take too much credit. Though I encouraged it, this is also just the way she came out. When she was a toddler, certain parts of her solid personality became particularly challenging. She made it abundantly clear who could hold her and for how long (spoiler alert—me, and me all the time). There was an entire year when she only wanted to wear purple! For a while there were seriously only five foods she decidedly liked. She was asserting herself and testing me with a strong opinion on just about everything. As hard as it was working with this fiery tot, I realized this tenacity of hers would serve her well later in life, so I never wished it away. Okay, maybe sometimes. But you get what I'm saying!

One of the most important qualities I aim to foster in my daughter is self-

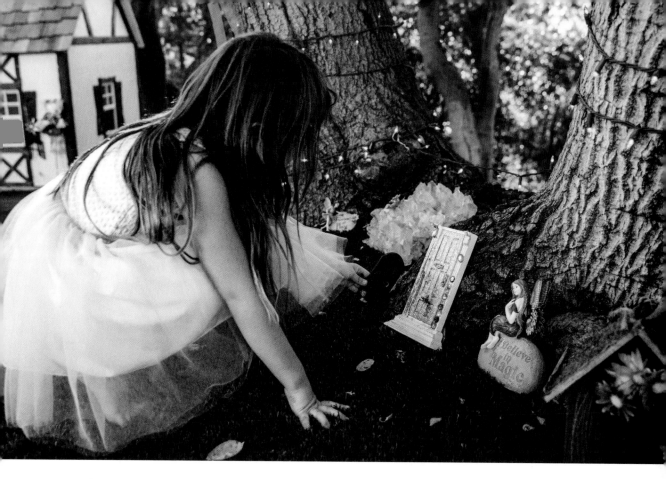

confidence. In the past five years as a parent I've learned that with little girls and kids in general, much of their confidence comes from knowing who they are and feeling good about that. I know having a solid sense of self will really come into play not only on the playground but throughout Evie's life when it comes to fitting in and making friends. At any age, knowing and liking the person we are helps us make better decisions, establish relationships, and feel good overall. I want my daughter to feel confident in expressing her strong opinions, even as a five-year-old. However, while I let Evie be her assertive self, I do lots of work not to let her think she rules our household. She is the type of kid who has to have very clear boundaries. Every time I forget that, she reminds me immediately. And knowing that about her helps me to set her up to succeed more in life.

When it comes to the two of us, the respect goes both ways. I've learned about the importance of listening and connecting to Evie before suddenly shifting gears on her. For example, when we get home and it's time to sit down for dinner, rather than pulling her from whatever it is she's into, I will take five minutes to connect with her, whether it means playing a quick game or drawing a picture. It takes only five short minutes for me to get on her level and make that connection. It's then much easier to say, "Let's go have some dinner," because she's had time to connect and transition. Sitting down to dinner becomes less of an order or demand and more of a natural flow of events. I feel this is a helpful tactic with the new age kids we are raising, who are independent minded and super opinionated. I had to ask my mom to be sure, but I definitely don't remember ever having the kind of strong

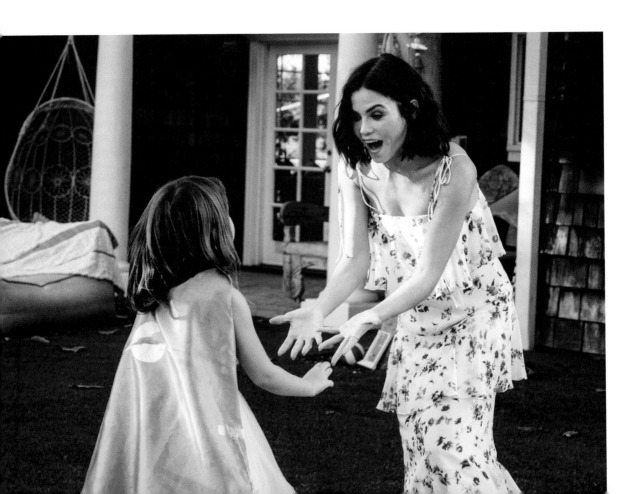

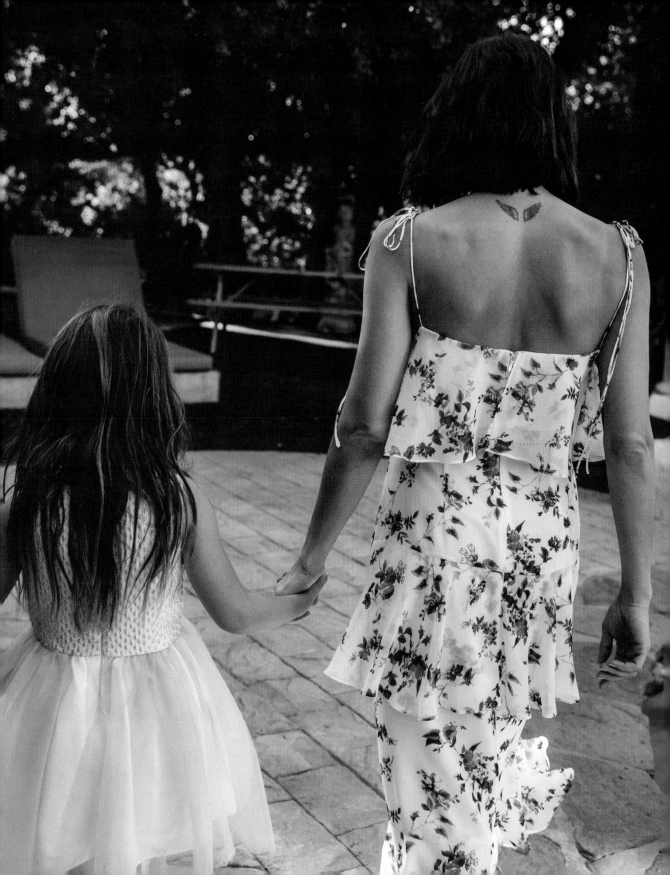

will Evie has. (My mom has confirmed I was much more easygoing. Grandmother amnesia? We will never know!)

The other day Evie and I went to the movies with some of her friends and their parents. We were in the elevator, when the doors opened on the wrong floor. When Evie began to step out, one of the other kids grabbed Evie's hand to stop her from exiting. Evie whipped around and hollered, "Don't tell me what to do!" as she pulled her arm back. Everyone in the elevator was stunned at the big reaction coming from this little person. It was intense! As her mom, even I was taken aback. *Okay, that just happened.* Once we were alone in the car I asked Evie what her reaction was all about. She proudly explained, "I don't need anybody to tell me what to do. I can handle myself. I'm a strong girl." *OH WOW.* In that moment I thought, *I've either done something so right or we have quite the future ahead of us. Possibly both.* Either way, it's pretty incredible that at such a young age she was thinking, *I can handle this. I would have figured out it was the wrong floor. And nobody can grab my arm and spin me around.* I like that about her and I hope this inner strength always sticks. This self-assured independence will certainly serve her in the future.

For little girls, confidence is all about feeling heard, being able to have an opinion, and not being told they have to be perfect all the time. In order to foster this sense of strength in my daughter I constantly get on her level. I act silly, get messy, and have fun, too! Instead of staying in mom mode, I take on a childlike mind-set in order to discover new ways I can engage with Evie and encourage her to expand her connection to nature and herself. One thing we've always done ever since she was an infant is free dance our hearts out. Dancing is one of the first things babies want to do. You can see their little spirits light up as they kick and bounce to music. It's a primal reaction: they can't help themselves, and it's so cute! Free dancing starts early on, so I say keep it going! It's a simple way to get children of all ages to connect to their

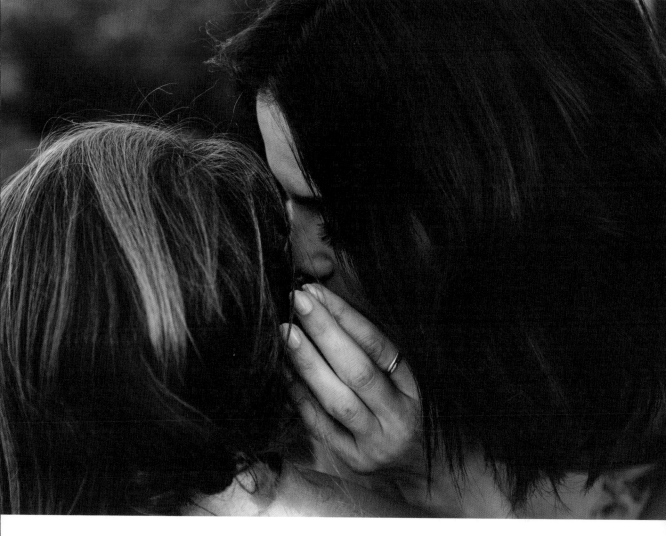

bodies, learn coordination and agility, and have fun. Not to mention it's a great way to release endorphins and relieve stress.

Much like me, Evie has rituals meant to guide her toward being her best self. She just doesn't realize that's what they are. Rather than merely entertain her and keep her busy, I hope through these practices to foster creativity, empathy, imagination,

and confidence. While they take some extra work on my part, I find them to be far more beneficial for her than plugging into an iPad.

organized chaos

Much like free dance, free art creates space for self-expression, creativity, and connection. I want my daughter to play, create, and not be afraid to draw outside the lines.

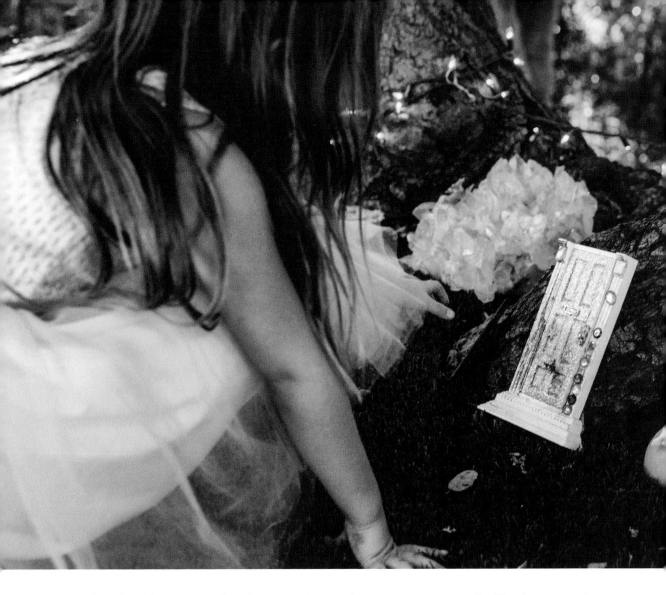

Unlike a lot of parents, I allow her to make a mess and experiment with glue or paint. A lot of moms might be cringing right now, but not to worry, I keep things confined in order to protect my house from turning into one big piece of purple glitter.

When we bought our current house, there was a very small office between the kitchen and the living room. A home office wasn't something we needed at the time, so we decided to give the room to Evie. Her dad and I had this idea to create a free art room where she could get really messy and do whatever she wanted in the name of art, as long as it was confined to this room. In there you'll find every kind of ingredient imaginable to make something with. You name a craft item and it's probably in there. What began as a blank slate has become a beautiful mess. The walls are painted. The floors are painted. Every inch and every crevice is covered with Evie's creativity. She goes in there to play on her own or we'll often go in there together. Play is the way kids connect with adults. If you want to connect more with your child, play more! We've made many castles out of toothpicks, paint, glitter glue, and cotton balls. Sometimes we'll just go in there and say, "Let's create something!" Fallen pine cones become sparkling paperweights. Dried leaves can be turned into stamps. She sees something now and thinks, *Oh, I can turn this into that!* I love how this type of activity activates that creative side of kids' brains.

You don't need to have a spare room in order to incorporate free art into your child's life. Sometimes I'll take an old sheet outside to create a special space for art activity. If you haven't done this before, you'll notice how excited your kids will be because they've been given permission to make a mess. And even if all Evie has made is a big ol' mess, I will find something to praise. I feel it's important for kids to have the opportunity to be carefree, whether it's through dance, art, or imagination. Their confidence soars when they feel clever, inventive, and creative.

the why train

Most parents or caretakers understand the annoyance of the why-why-why. "No, you can't go to the store without pants on." *Why?* "No, we can't buy thirty packs of gum." *Why?* The why train takes off when kids are around four or five years old. Although responding "Because I said so" can be kind of fun because that's what most of us were told, I don't believe it's necessarily the right answer. Besides, I don't think it ever really works. I believe in answering the *why?* instead of stopping it in its tracks. The biggest reason is that I respect Evie and her thoughts. I want her to always feel free to ask me questions. In order to instill the habit of asking why, I have to be willing to answer it myself. When Evie gets on a *why* train I think, *All right, let's see where this thing goes.* I'll answer her *why?*, which usually leads to the next *why?*, and then the next. It's an opportunity for me to understand how her mind works. The questions she asks are very indicative of how she feels and how she processes the world around her. It's also a great challenge for me! Sometimes I don't know the answer and I'll have to find out for her. Overall it's a great bonding opportunity and a chance for us to learn together.

I always want Everly to ask herself, others, and the universe *why?* I like to think of the *why* as a shovel: it's how we dig deeper.

mystical play

I've always encouraged Evie to believe in magic. I want my daughter, like myself, to have faith in something bigger than her in a way she can understand and relate to. She's always loved the idea of a magical, unseen presence, which in recent years has become a strong belief in fairies. She is absolutely fairy obsessed.

I fully support Evie's fairy fantasies because they're important to her. They have become part of our landscape and daily rituals. We placed a small plastic door meant for a dollhouse under a tree (aka the Fairy Tree) in our front yard. Evie believes this door leads to a magical world where the fairies live. She leaves them notes and they (ahem, I) leave her notes and sweet treats in return. It creates a sense of joy and innocence I want her to maintain for as long as possible. Ev believes there's a fairy for everything. There's the "I went to bed on time" fairy and the "I did a great job at the dentist" fairy. It's a great morning when she wakes up next to a note from the "good night's sleep" fairy! I figure, what's wrong with believing? And let me tell you, mamas, these fairies can be quite useful at times! The "I stayed in my bed all night long" fairy has visited quite a few times! It makes her happy, reinforces good choices, and gives her confidence. I also love the idea of her

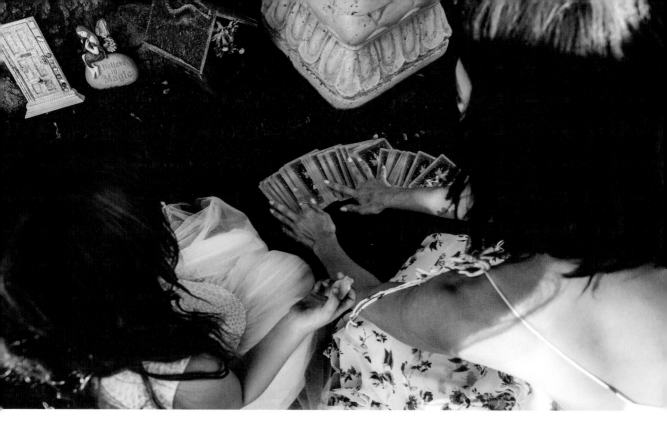

believing in a certain mystical, magical way of life and knowing there's a special energy all around us, whatever you want to name it, because I do, too. This mystical mind-set has created a beautiful spiritual bond for us.

respect your mother (earth, that is!)

One of the most important tasks for a modern-day mom is making sure our kids are connecting to nature. From a very young age, kids today have so much interest in technology. They have access to television, smartphones, tablets, and so forth. There are endless external stimuli coming at our kids, and avoiding them is pretty much impossible. Getting back to the basics is more important now than ever. This doesn't mean Evie can't have an iPad or that I don't allow her to enjoy movies or shows. I want her to experience those things as well. But to counterbalance them, I do put extra effort into creating a relationship between her and nature. For us, this can mean anything from visiting the ocean, going on nature walks, camping, or even keeping it close to home and playing in the backyard. Sometimes we lie in the grass, looking up at the clouds and trying to find shapes of familiar things. With all the latest apps and games out there, one might assume kids would be bored by these sort of activities, but I've found that Evie and her friends respond really well. As a result, Evie knows how special trees, flowers, and plants are. And she understands the importance of being good to nature because I make it a point to lead by example by recycling, picking up litter, and talking about how we can be better to our mother earth. One of her favorite sayings is, "Fairies like glitter but they don't like litter!" Because she respects nature she is very upset by litter. It makes me proud knowing the planet is in better hands with kids like Evie looking after it!

roses and thorns game

When it comes to bedtime, Evie will do anything and everything she can to put off actually going to bed. She can identify the one thing she forgot that happens to be on the other side of the house, or maybe the blanket covering her is just not feeling right. It's a spectacular show she puts on, one that amazes me every time. I've learned that during this time I can basically ask her anything to retrieve any information I want, because she will do anything it takes to keep me in that room. In light of this charade, I decided to turn the go-to-bed game into an opportunity to connect with my girl.

I'll ask her every night, "What was your rose and what was your thorn from today?" The rose will be the best part, the highlight of her day. And the thorn will be the part of her day she didn't feel the greatest about. This helps Evie evaluate her emotions by connecting to herself. I make it a point just to listen, not to try and fix anything for her. If she were to say the thorn was when someone at school was mean to her, I would show my empathy and understanding by simply saying, "That must have been hurtful." This conversation fosters a sweeter, deeper connection between us. It's a nice little moment to have with each other and a lovely way to end every day.

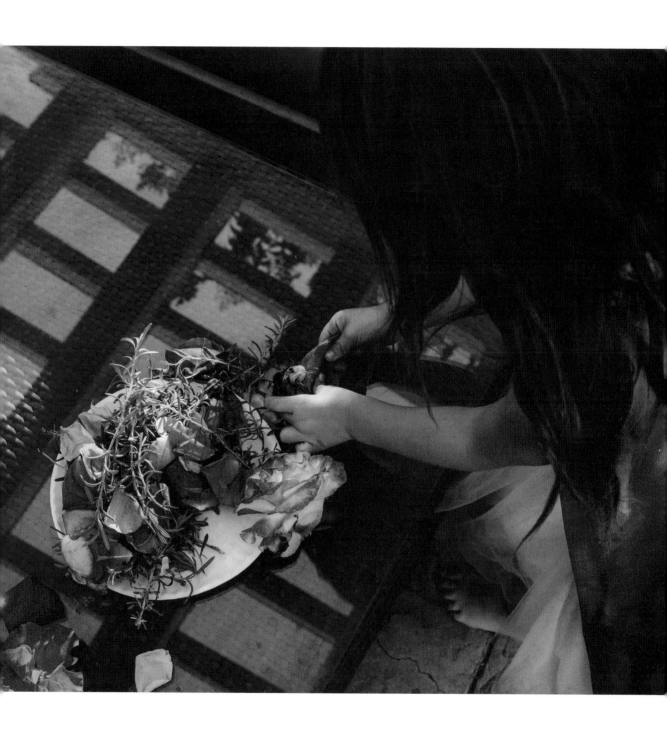

TAKE WITH YOU

When it comes to parenting, I have learned there is no one way,
no right way! No matter how many people give you advice or how
many books you read, the best compass for what is best for your
child is inside of you. Your own gut instinct is almost always right.
My doula, Joanne, taught me this. I would go through moments of
second-guessing or being too hard on myself as a mother. I overly
researched topics I didn't necessarily have to. And I often wondered
if Evie was acting differently from other kids and if she was, was it
my fault? Was I doing everything "right"? My doula finally said to me
that I needed to relax and listen to myself more. She said, "You are
very sure of yourself as a woman. You know what you value, and you
know how to love. That is all you need." And when it came time for
any big milestones like weaning from breastfeeding, sleep training
versus not sleep training, pacifier removal, you name it . . . every time
I found myself in the struggle of *What should I do?*, I reminded
myself of what Joanne said and learned to trust what I knew within.

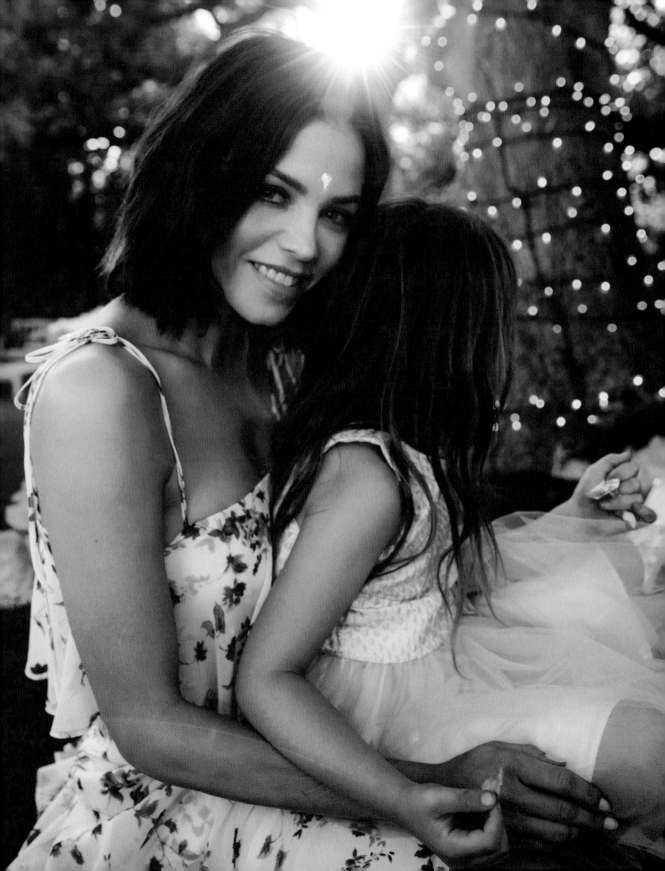

Heartbreak

The most startling thing about heartbreak is in the
looking back and noticing that the world didn't
actually end.

— APRIL GREEN

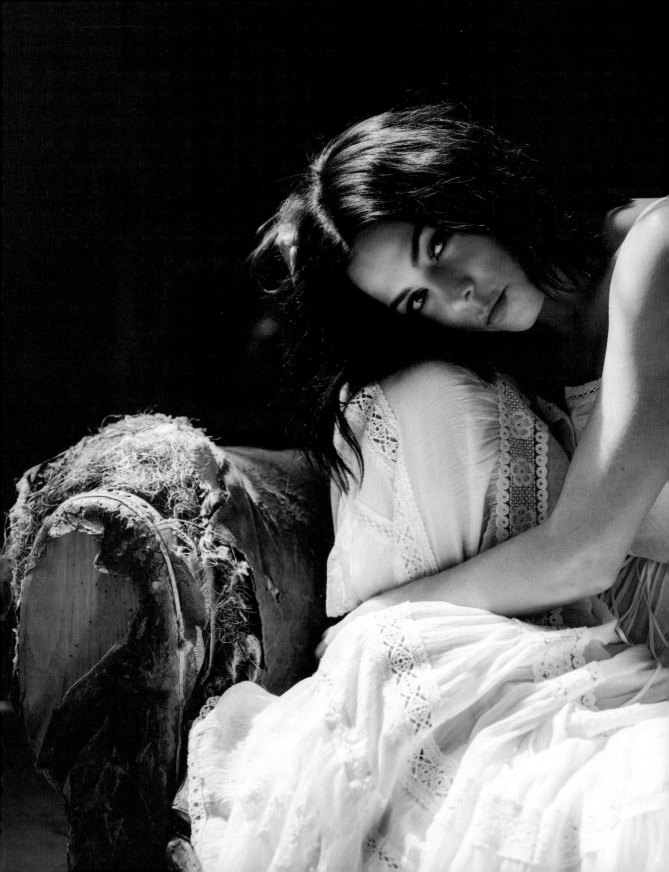

CHAPTER NINE

gracefully you

To say I've learned a thing or two in the past year would be the understatement of my life. I didn't realize the true meaning of strength, resilience, and grace until I went through a major life change—in the public eye, too. Nobody who sets out to get married ever wants a divorce. I certainly didn't. One thing I know for sure, no matter the why or how, it's still very hard to go through the process of separation regardless of your situation. During that time of change, you see certain characteristics you wish you didn't see in the other person. It was a hard truth for me to realize that the relationship I was in hadn't evolved as we had as individuals. That I had grown, and seen the light of myself, so to speak. I wasn't certain how one should deal with that truth. I sat with mine for a while, unsure of what to do. I always talk about people empowering themselves, encouraging others to live their truth. For me not to walk my talk wasn't an option. I didn't want to be inauthentic to what I was outwardly all about. I needed to find my own inner strength in order to practice what I'd preached.

So I faced the music of my marriage. Where we were as a couple. Where I was as a woman. I'd come to realize the dynamic I was in wasn't serving me, nor was it serving my daughter. It wasn't serving anyone, really. First and foremost, I had to accept the realization that this wasn't working and had moved into hurting. It was a painful, scary place for me to sit and ponder. I wondered, *How am I going to deal with this gracefully?* I knew it wouldn't be pretty or perfect in any way, no matter what I did or didn't do. But if every day throughout the process I woke up and decided I was going to be my best self, rise above the fray, and elevate my intentions as much as possible—not only for myself but for Everly, too—we could all hopefully move forward with dignity and grace.

I've always been a very, positive person. When pain jabbed me hard and deep in the past, I'd take the easy way out by planning an escape or orchestrating a distraction in order to press fast-forward and seemingly keep myself happy. The problem with this strategy is that it never really works. The pain will always linger in some way because it was never properly dealt with or put to rest. I didn't want that to be the case this time, so I decided not to run away from what was happening but rather to deal with it head-on. Facing your pain means moving into a more candid place of being. It's looking at the issue at hand directly in the eyes and saying, *I see you. I'm not going to run away from you. Let's do this.* It involves a lot of listening to yourself,

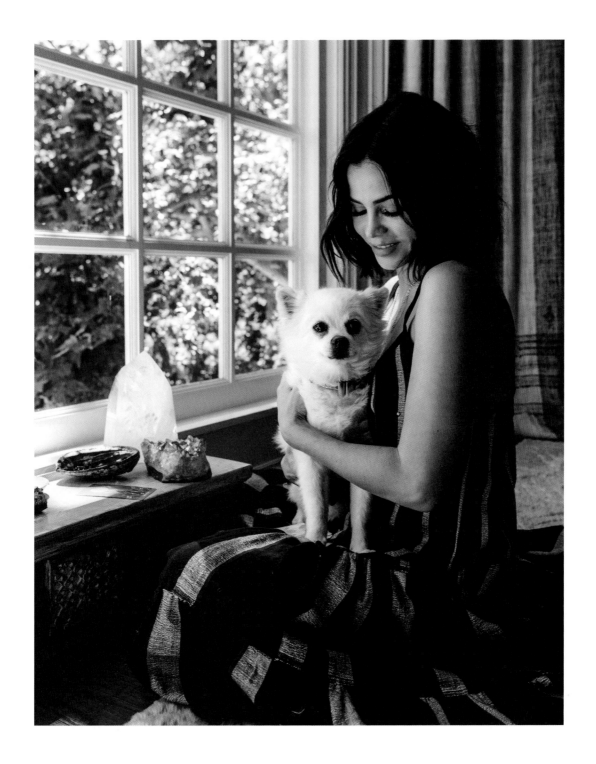

honoring your boundaries, and working through your feelings as they show up. It's allowing yourself to cry, scream, and sob when you need it as opposed to bury your feelings and move forward. I couldn't fly above or dig below the darkness this time around. The only way was to go right through the tunnel in order to get to the light. This route was extremely difficult for me. I didn't want to face my sadness. It wasn't the route I wanted to take, but it was the best way for me to go. I reminded myself of that every day, over and over again. Focusing on the light at the other side of the harrowing darkness helped me make it through. It also taught me a huge life lesson in what it means to find my grace.

In the beginning of my separation, it felt as though I were in a dark closet, desperately trying to find the light or the way out. I was in a state of shock. The phases I went through contrasted starkly. One week I'd be doing really well and the next I was slammed with a whole slew of emotions. The last thing I wanted to do was project emotionally, reacting all over the place. The rumor mill was churning out story after story. There were many times I hid under the covers, wondering what was next. The pain hit me like a tumbling avalanche. I was completely overcome with fear and sadness. It took many moments of my sitting alone with my grief to force me into surrendering to my roller coaster of a situation.

Eventually I was able to take a step back for a bird's-eye view of where my life was at. Putting everything into perspective got me to a place of acceptance, where I could say, *Okay, I am on this roller coaster but I'm not going to let it define me or allow myself to get out of control.* I decided I was not going to allow myself to feel as though I was at the mercy of my life. While I didn't have control over what was going on around me, I did and always will have control over my choices and actions. I took a social media break and swore to myself not to read whatever the online opinions would be. Then, after initial heavy grief, an interesting thing

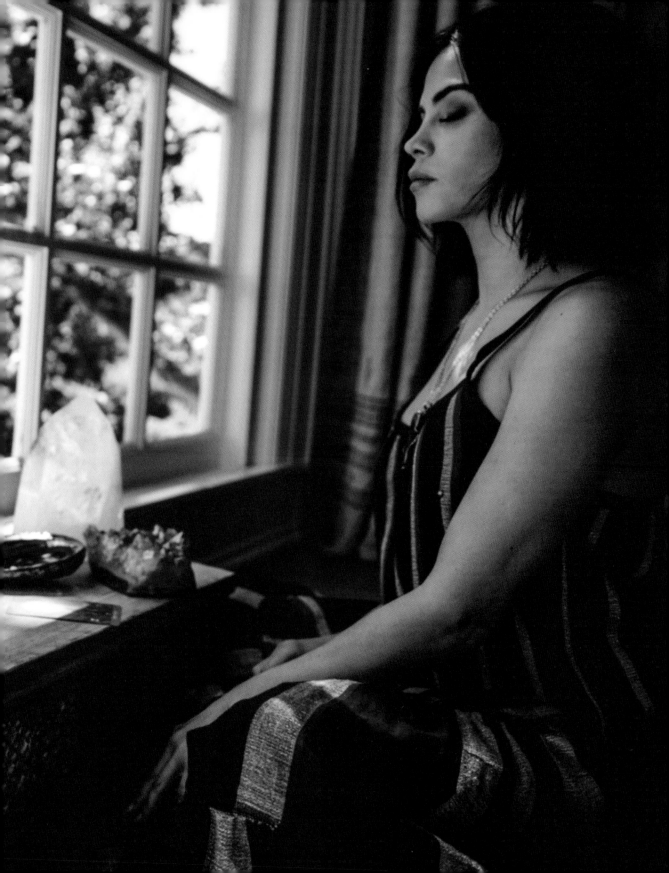

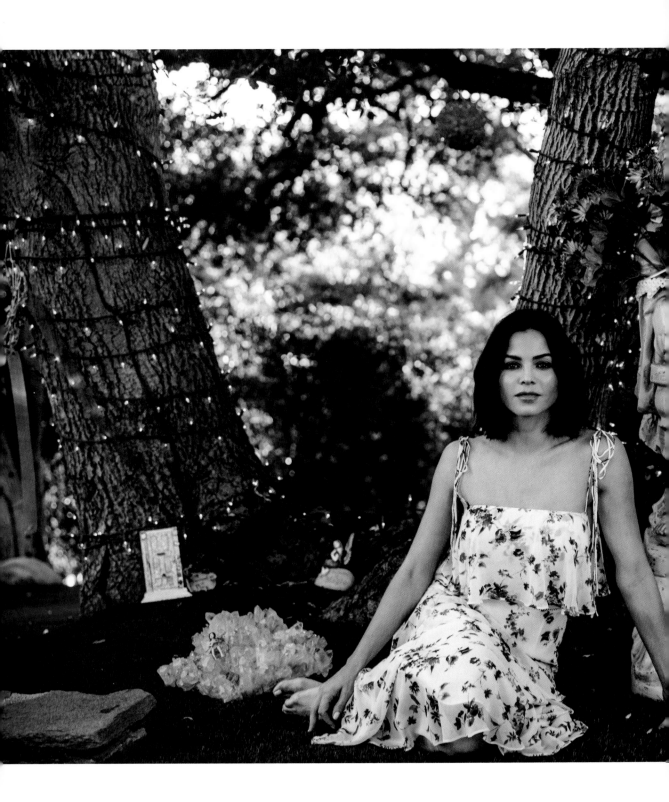

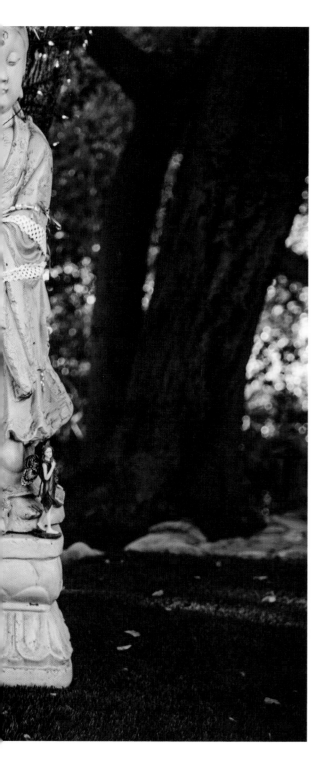

happened. Everything lightened up. I felt free. Free of heavy emotions and situations I had been carrying around like a bag of bricks for far too long. I felt inspired by my strength. Very shortly after the separation was announced, I was thrust into doing press for *World of Dance*. At first I was overwhelmed by the prospect of being asked about my personal life, but soon enough realized I felt lighter, happier . . . okay. I was okay. I felt all the support and love coming from the world.

It was a lesson for me in remembering to allow for divine surprise in life. You think you know how everything will go. Will feel. And then life delights you with unexpected grace. I was really grateful for that. The decision to act, live, and accept grace kept me from emotionally exploding on social media or otherwise acting inappropriately in a way I'd later regret.

What is grace to me? We all feel our absolute best when we are acting as our best selves. Every day we are presented with opportunities, through the choices we make, the words we use, and the actions we take, to make conscious decisions on how we go about living. Grace is the feeling we get from living our greatest potential. It's a calm breath, an expanded sigh. Fear, on the other hand, is the antithesis of grace. It's a heated, contracted space we feel trapped in when we resort to things like blame or retaliation. Blaming is one of the most ungraceful things one can do. Spewing all your bad feelings onto another person doesn't get you anywhere. It also makes people not want to be around you because they'll feel bad. You've become a toxic vortex people avoid, not wanting to be dragged into your bad place. The only people who will stick around are miserable ones, because misery loves company. And who wants to be surrounded by misery? Not me. It's okay to be sad and to acknowledge those emotions, but to make somebody else sad is simply ungraceful.

GRACEFUL PAIN

At times it was tempting for me to act out. I'm human, after all. Plus I was sometimes forced into a defensive position. However, I really wanted to prove to myself that I could move through pain and hardship by making choices based on my highest potential. This is especially hard to do in the moment, when you're not expecting someone you love to act a certain way or cause you pain. You're hit with that harsh reality, and then what do you do? Do you act out? Hit back? The instinct is to lash out or project onto the other person. This works for us momentarily, and sometimes it needs to happen. There's no shame in that game. But the best way to move beyond anguish is by becoming a bigger, better person. This means instead of immediately reacting, internalizing the situation by asking, *What is this situation saying about me?* Pain will always show you that. If you can see the conflict as a lesson, adopt that sort of mentality, and get yourself out of the blame game, then you will move forward every time.

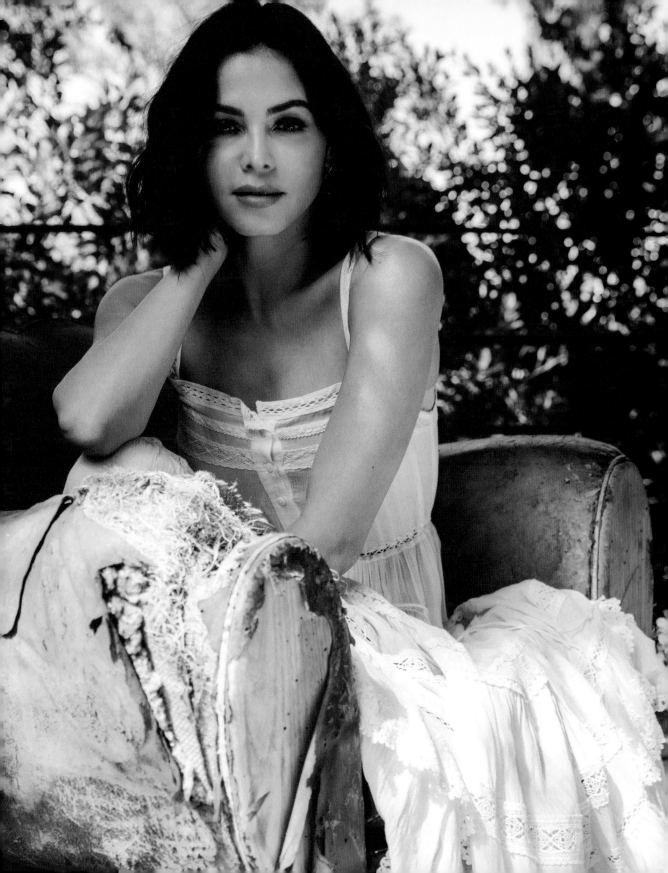

For me, it was so important to first hit pause and find the grace. I had to reel myself in every day, taking a moment to remind myself not to react right away. I'd then allow myself to feel the pain from a hit, honor my feelings, and go through a process of acceptance. Like, *Okay, that just happened. Now what?* Once I worked through it internally, I felt lighter and less fired up. From that place I could then react. This way of dealing with things is really about honoring yourself. Some days are easier than others. Being graceful means reminding yourself of your true intentions regardless of who said what about you. It is letting go of things that are not meant for you. It is knowing when to move on from people who don't belong in your life. Acting with grace is easy to do when life is good and things are going your way. The real challenge is when you're pushed past your boundaries and feel you've lost your footing in life. That's when the work begins and when it matters most.

The separation storm tested me in ways I hadn't thought possible. I started to wonder if everything I believed in and always talked about was even real. Could anyone or anything ever be trusted? Was there a light at the end of the tunnel? How could I be so sure? I slowly started to see the light break through as I made my way to the other side. And one day I realized—the light is there! And it's more than just light! The other side was dazzling with luck, joy, and a happiness my mind couldn't have conjured up or even comprehended before I embarked on this soul-searching journey. The best part is, I had it all within me the whole time. I had to live in it and go through it in order to accept that this is how life works. I found a bigger, more expanded part of myself along with a new basis for life. I even found deep love with someone new, deeper than I had imagined before. I couldn't have come to this place without fully trusting and wholly surrendering to grace.

In the end, I realized I could view every hardship as an opportunity to learn about myself. Rather than getting stuck in the muck of my own misery, I should embrace it. Trust that everything happens for a reason and there will be a beautiful lesson somewhere in there. When something or someone goes awry, think, don't do. I'll begin by asking myself, *What is this showing me that I need to change?* Processing teaches us a massively valuable lesson about ourselves. Without pain, friction, and contrast, we wouldn't grow, so take it as an opportunity. By living this way, you're learning about yourself and therefore evolving positively. As a result, you'll draw like-minded people toward you, ones who match this higher vibration level you're living on. You'll also attract elevated situations to your work, home, and love life. I discovered that when you choose to focus on your growth while being your own biggest cheerleader, you will rise above the challenges and find the grace. You will create a better life for yourself all around.

GIRL GRACE

One of the most profound and surprising lessons I've learned about acting with grace came from an unexpected place:

Channing's ex-girlfriend. Before he and I met, Channing was in a long-term relationship with a woman named Erica. They'd lived a whole life with each other before I came along, even moving to LA together to pursue his acting career. I thought about her a lot early on because Chan and I connected very soon after they'd broken up. At that point, *Step Up* was exploding everywhere. My heart ached for her whenever I'd imagine what it must have been like processing the loss of your longtime love while every billboard, magazine, and commercial featured a smoldering photo of your ex with his new girlfriend. Even though I didn't know her, I hated knowing I was that person for her. I'm not here for women against women, old versus new. Even though it made no difference in my life, I really hoped she didn't hold resentment toward me.

One night on my way into an event at the Four Seasons hotel, I walked straight into Erica for the first time. I was so nervous and anxious about what she might say or do to me, the new girl. Women can be emotional—we all know this to be true. To my utter surprise, Erica couldn't have been more gracious. She stopped to say hello, giving me the biggest smile and hug, showing genuine kindness. I'm sure on some level it was shocking and a little painful for her. It would have been for me. I imagine there was a small part of her that wanted to walk on by and ignore me, but you'd never have known it. There was no snarky attitude whatsoever. She was all grace. Erica chose to be loving and supportive when she could have been horrible. She didn't have to be lovely or address me at all. I can't say for sure I would have been as gracious as Erica had the roles been reversed. I'm willing to bet the way this interaction played out felt better and brought a level of closure for her. She didn't have to go home feeling like, *Aw, man, I lowered myself to that level.* We've all experienced that next-day regret after acting impulsively in a way of which we aren't proud. She also didn't have to worry about running into me again, because we all survived. It didn't have to be an awkward or bad thing.

This situation stuck with me for so long. It was that powerful for me. Our two-minute interaction showed me how possible it is to live in this higher vibration. Grace is an ever-present force we can tap into when we need it. It's having wisdom ahead of you so you can always take the high road. This can be difficult in the moment, but in the end you—and everyone else—will always walk away feeling better than when you arrived.

VIRAL GRACE

I remember one day I was in the worst mood and just feeling really over life. I was hunting around a drugstore when I noticed this woman. She was frazzled, struggling to get through the store with her two kids, who were running around being wild. She caught my eye and looked at me with this truly sweet smile. Her whole demeanor changed as she beamed and exclaimed, "Oh, I love watching you on TV! *Witches of East End* is my favorite show! The best part of the week!" Her happiness and excitement were contagious. They pulled me out of my own funk. If this crazed, struggling mother could flip her own switch like that, so could I. Our encounter changed my whole day around. That's the power of love and grace.

Imagine how much kinder the world would be if everyone chose to be the grace in someone else's day. I think about this a lot when I'm driving. Here in LA, people tend to be very aggressive behind the wheel. When someone cuts me off and flips me off in traffic (hey, it happens), it takes a real effort for me not to return the middle finger or obnoxiously honk my horn. But what good will that do? If I take on their bad mood, I'll likely project it onto someone else, allowing the lack of grace to spread like wildfire. Their attitude stops with them. Same goes for everywhere else: the grocery store, the bank, the coffee shop. We've all had to deal with a disgruntled person hustling us along because they're in a mood. Rather than mirroring their darkness, try showing them some light. You never know how badly their day has gone. Maybe they're working through something really difficult like a sick parent or financial depression.

Be the grace in their day by showing them kindness. Pay them a compliment or leave them with a smile. There's not a single person, not even the most pessimistic person in the world, who doesn't want to feel good.

COMPLIMENT CHALLENGE

To keep myself on track in terms of spreading positivity, someone gave me the idea to give at least three organic compliments a day. Not only does it feel like a fun game, it also encourages me to look for light throughout the day. I'll notice things I might otherwise walk right by without acknowledging their greatness. But mostly, I know I'm making others feel my light by shining it their way. If I see a stranger with great style, I'll let them know. When I hear someone humming to themselves in the grocery store I'll tell them, *That's my jam, too.* Life's too short not to connect with those around you!

CLEAR THE FEAR

People try to write their own stories all the time. When fear creeps in, we tell

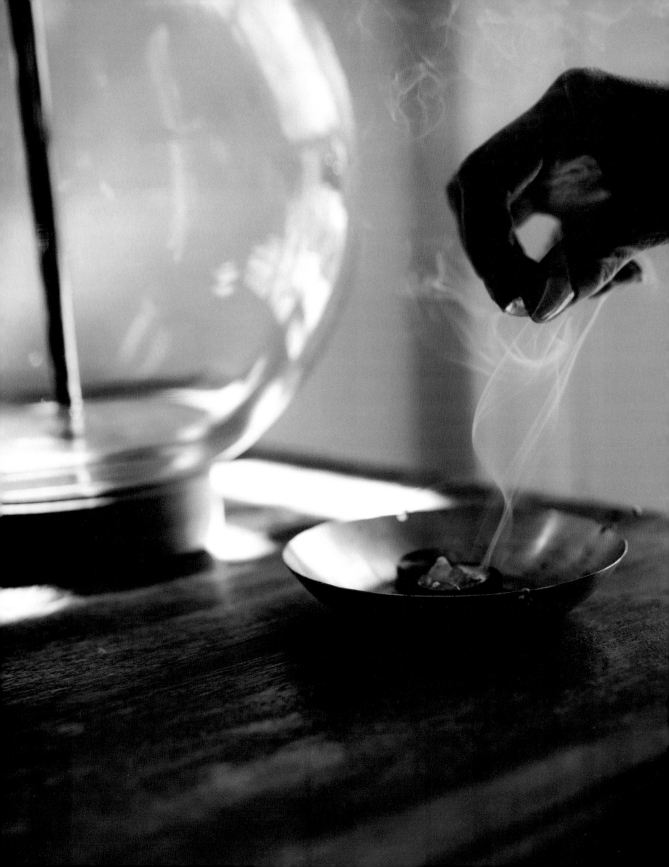

ourselves things like, *This is going to be so bad*, or *I'm never going to find love again—nobody will every love me like this person*. Grace is that energy that comes in and says, *How about you sit back and stop trying to write your own story?*

There was a point before Channing and I announced our separation where I thought, *How in the world will everyone handle this?* The public had known us as a couple forever, and not just a couple—the perfect couple. How would people at work react when I went in the next day? Would they pity me? Assume the worst had happened? I was scared of everything that would follow our coming out.

On top of that pressure were my fears of moving forward. What would that look like? Dating . . . ? Then there was my daughter. She's very shy and funny and standoffish with men. It takes her a long time to warm up to others. I predicted this child was going to be so jealous of whoever else I spent time with. How would I ever date with her blessing? My fears were going haywire. *The world is going to freak*

out. My daughter is going to freak out. I am totally freaking out. At the end of the day I just kept telling myself to trust, trust, trust. And trust I did. The news of our divorce didn't drown me. Not to any extent I couldn't handle, anyway. When I was ready, I started dating someone amazing. It was this cosmically great thing where we circled back around toward each other after a moment of instant recognition years ago. Those stories you hear of seeing someone and feeling an instant remembrance that just sticks with you? Well, I had it happen, despite the odds. (Cheers to you, universe!) Lo and behold, everything started flowing together. Evie has embraced her new normal with a great amount of ease. It all came together in a truly graceful way.

Just when you think you've written your own story and you know how it's going to go, you have to allow for that serious element of grace and divinity. There are going to be things good and bad that you didn't see coming, but there's always a rhyme or reason to them. Fear is what happens when we think we're handling everything on our own. Grace is there to step in and say, *Let me handle this.* Trusting in the universe and grace is something we have to do action by action, intention by intention. It's a practice like everything else. Little miracles happen every day. Believe in them and they'll happen to you!

THE GRACE MUSCLE

Listen, I was never challenged by anything more than I was by having to find grace during my divorce. Not only was I fighting an emotional battle of having to let go and move forward in life, I was learning things about my ex most people wouldn't have to face—and over the internet, as it was happening. There I was, on a plane, alone, finding out about his new relationship. I felt blindsided. Choosing grace as I learned everything about my personal situation along with the rest of the world was really difficult. It was quite a challenge to remain graceful, to say the least. That's when your real character comes out. Instead of reacting the

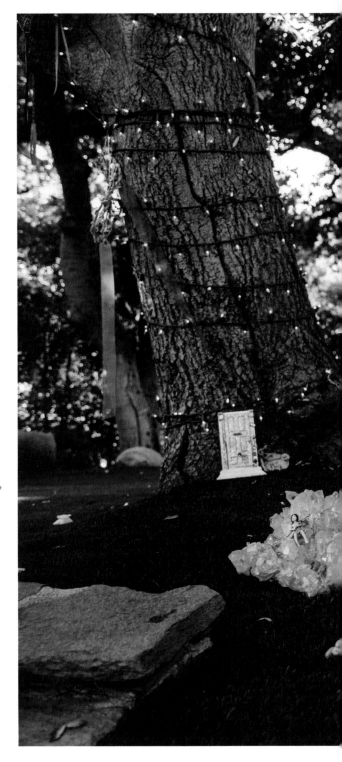

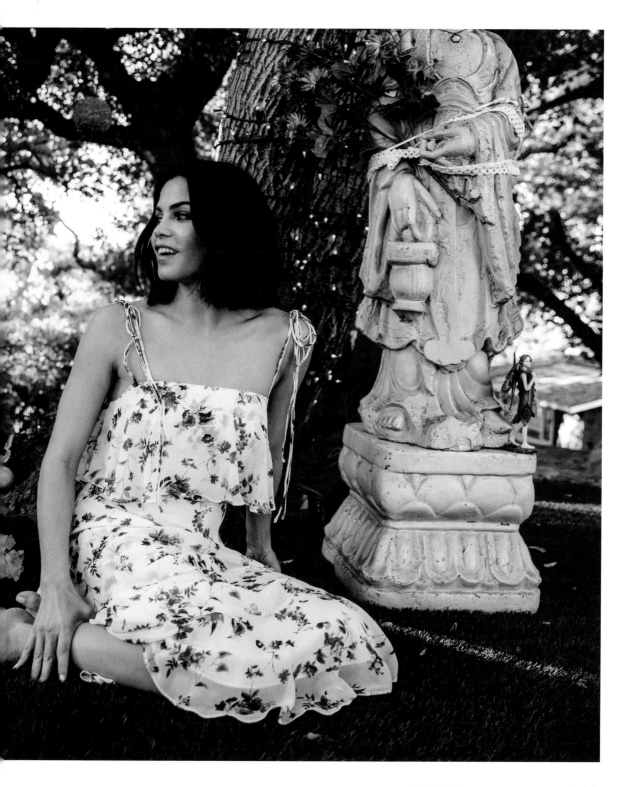

way I wanted to (there were many Twitter posts written, then deleted—more on that below), I asked myself this: *How do I choose grace in this moment?* Had I not been practicing this way of life beforehand, I definitely wouldn't have handled this news very gracefully. I've decided grace is like a muscle. When you use it every day, you're building strength to stay on a higher level. By keeping it strong and toned, you make sure it's there for you whenever you need it.

GET OVER THE OVERSHARE

Before the days of social media, people in the public eye could hide behind their publicists, waiting out any type of tabloid storm. These days, everyone has smartphones, and they're waiting to see what you're going to say, right off the cuff. I believe Twitter is fun but can be a very dangerous tool. It invites impulsive behavior, allowing us to say what we want to say in that moment without careful consideration of what we're putting out there. Do you know how many

times I've wanted to go online and write exactly what's on my mind? Thousands. I receive countless tweets coming at me containing misconceptions, lies, or hurtful comments. My instinct is to fight back, set the record straight. What stops me every time is the thought, *Choose to say what you would want yourself to live with a week from today.* Or, when the stakes are really high, *Choose what you would want Everly to read when she's older.* I want both her and myself to be proud of my choices. We all have the strength of mind to not let ourselves overreact.

I have many, many drafts of tweets I wanted to send out, but instead I saved them and deleted them. It's sort of like a social media journal consisting of unsent tweets. The modern-day equivalent of writing a letter and burning it. My "write it, save it, delete it" method can be applied to every scenario. Mad at your boss? Write, save, delete. Pissed off at your boyfriend? Write, save, delete. We are in this crazy time where everyone has the ability to stand on a soapbox and project. As they say, the internet is forever. We should all choose our words wisely, whether we have forty followers or four million.

SIGNS OF GRACE

The universe is brimming with signs. All we have to do is keep an open heart and an open mind in order to see and receive them. Signs are always showing up for me, moments where little things show up along my path. I really hold on to signs when I witness them because I know it means I'm going in the right direction. Often someone I need to connect with will call me at exactly the right time. Or I'll choose to go with friends to a place I've never been before and I'll meet people there who mirror where I want to be going in life. Things seem to really roll out when you go with the flow, follow the signs, and allow life to show you what it has in store for you.

TAKE WITH YOU

Grace and the universe go hand in hand. When I'm feeling especially open and expanded, I'll get a lot of people commenting, "You really look lighter." And it's because I feel lighter, happier, more graceful. Whenever I'm feeling stuck and at the mercy of life, I get out more to see what's possible. That's when signs seem to really show up. Oftentimes I'll say, *Had I not been at this place at this time, I wouldn't have been available for this extraordinary thing to happen.* Show up for possibility, and the universe will always show up for you.

gracefully now

i began writing this book in the midst of the craziest year of my life. I went through a divorce, lost my beloved dog, Lulu, of eleven years, and stood by the side of one of my best friends as she lost her battle with cancer and crossed over. It was definitely a year of grief and challenges for me. But it was a year of joyful surprises as well. I learned this: you never know what you're capable of or the level of strength you carry within you until you've been challenged to go beyond your limits of comfort and familiarity.

You, too, can face any challenges that come your way. The opportunity to show up for yourself will arise. Although it may be painful and difficult, you can and will come out on the other side a stronger, more expanded, better version of yourself. To achieve this, you'll need two things: work and trust.

I wish I could say at the conclusion of this book that everything in my life has fallen into place and all is perfect now, but the truth is, life is a process. As long as we're here, there are always going to be challenges. Just when I thought it was all smooth sailing, Evie and I received notice that we had only twenty-four hours to move out of our house (thank you, mold!). Despite having the rug pulled out from under us (literally!), we managed to turn moving into an adventure. Sometimes I sit alone with my thoughts and look around, and even in the thick of chaos and uncertainty I think, *Life is still getting better.* It doesn't mean there won't be hardships ahead or challenges around the corner, but now that I've been through some really tough stuff I have a strong faith in knowing we all survive and only improve and get better. And every single experience that happens to you is an opportunity for growth.

Trust life. Love yourself. After the rain, there is always a rainbow.

I have so many people to thank for helping me bring this vision to life! Thank you to Natasha, Hannah, and the great team at Simon & Schuster for supporting me from the very beginning and for putting up with my many last-minute thoughts, ideas, and changes!

Thank you to Cooking with Om for the nutritional yummy inspiration and all-around delicious help.

To my soul brother Brad Goreski. Thank you for always getting me, dancing with me, and being in my corner 100 percent. And boy, do we have fun . . . !

To Allie, my partner in crime. You are pure light and love and I can't thank you enough for your dedication and help with everything. You are pure heart and magic.

To Evelyn O'Neill and everyone at Management 360, as well as UTA, Nicole Perna, Jeffrey Chassen, Brett Ruttenberg, and Dave Feldman–it takes a village and you are my village. I thank you!

To my family, for loving me no matter what. Thank you for teaching me what unconditional love feels like so early on in my life. It's a gift of gratitude I will never be able to put into words!

To my love–you are the biggest gift in my life. You inspire me and make me stand in awe and thank my lucky stars every single day. I love you!

To Evie–you are my heart. This book is for you. I hope to make you proud every single day. Always remember to be true to yourself no matter what and shine that very special light of yours. I love you to infinity and beyond and always will!